CYNTHIA E. FINCHER, PHD

Healthy Living in a
Toxic World

Simple Ways to Protect Yourself & Your Family
from Hidden Health Risks

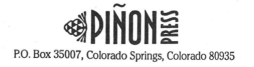

PIÑON PRESS

P.O. Box 35007, Colorado Springs, Colorado 80935

Library of Congress Catalog Card Number: 96-16483
ISBN 08910-99786

Fincher, Cynthia E.
    Healthy living in a toxic world : simple ways to
protect yourself and your family from hidden health risks
/ Cynthia E. Fincher
        p.   cm.
    Includes bibliographical references.
    1. Toxicology—Popular works. 2. Product safety.
    I. Title.
    RA1213.F49   1996
    615.9—dc20   96-16483
                                                    CIP

Printed in the United States of America

1 2 3 4 5 6 7 8 9 10 11 12 13 14 15 / 99 98 97 96

Contents

This book is lovingly dedicated to the two visionaries in my life:

In memory of my father, Forrest Gilbert Riecken,
a wise counselor, who encouraged me to set higher goals
and helped me reach them, and who taught by analogy.

And to my husband, Mark Edward Fincher,
the kindest and gentlest person I know,
who has supported and encouraged me,
and who has pondered with me about how to provide
a balanced perspective.

Preface

I remember hearing a newscast as a child that red dye in bubble gum had been shown to cause cancer in laboratory mice. I had a picture in my mind of rows and rows of cages holding laboratory mice blowing little pink bubbles. It all seemed ludicrous and unimportant. What kind of person would work to link a treat like bubble gum to some mystifying, terrifying death?

This is not a book about being afraid of cancer. It's a book about life. It's about living healthy and being free from the harm brought to all of us through the overuse of chemicals. It's about well people staying well.

For others, it's about solving the mystery behind the headaches, the fatigue, or the hyperactivity and poor health in their children. It's about people keeping alert minds and good memories for their entire lives.

Most of all, this book provides a framework in which the entire field of chemical usage, chemical research, and chemical warnings can be understood. It will enable people to make wise choices based on accurate knowledge. These choices will also significantly decrease the risk of cancer.

Acknowledgments

My husband, Mark Fincher, has been an invaluable source of help and inspiration on this project. He helped carry props to most of the seminars I taught, and he has read so many versions of the current manuscript that he may never read the actual book.

Marcia Findlay was important in moving this project from a seminar to a book by arranging the professional audio taping of this material and by her years of prayers and support.

I would like to thank Dr. Kim Kelly at the University of North Texas for her consultations on psychoneuroimmunology. I also appreciate all of the scientists, EPA officials, and professionals who gave phone interviews and sent their research.

I also appreciate the background I received from my parents in teaching and in counseling.

I would like to express appreciation to my editor, Traci Mullins, for her work to make the manuscript more interesting and easy to read.

CHAPTER ONE

IS THIS BOOK FOR YOU?

Have you ever wondered why so many people have chronic health problems?

Did you know that many of the household products sitting under your kitchen sink can cause headaches, fatigue, memory loss, irritability, depression, insomnia, vision problems, joint pain, nausea, and loss of coordination?

Toxic chemicals are so thoroughly ingrained into the fabric of our lives that only the well-informed even know which products contain them. Many of these toxic chemicals have seeped into our drinking water and live in our kitchen cabinets without warning labels or lists of potential side-effects. How often do we make the connection between their presence and a child's hyperactivity, a woman's chronic fatigue, or a grandparent's senility?

Toxic chemicals do not cause disease the way bacteria or viruses do, because toxic chemicals are not germs, they are poisons. Poisons accumulate in your body. If too much poison accumulates, it causes injury.

Toxic chemicals cause many kinds of injuries and diseases because they are able to travel throughout the body. For instance, a chemical injury to the DNA in your cells could lead to cancer or birth defects. A chemical injury to your brain could lead to Alzheimer's disease, Parkinson's disease, seizures, or depression. A chemical injury to your immune system could make you susceptible to every cold and flu virus that comes along or impair your ability to recover from it, or could make you vulnerable to autoimmune diseases.

A chemical injury to your cardiovascular system could lead to high blood pressure and increased risk of heart attack. A chemical injury to your digestive system could lead to nausea, loss of appetite, problems digesting food, or irritable bowel syndrome. A chemical injury to your endocrine system could lead to PMS, hypothyroidism, and an increased risk of breast cancer.

Other health conditions related to chemical injuries affect people in all age groups. We're seeing more and more cases of children with learning disabilities, attention deficits, and hyperactivity. Adults are being diagnosed with conditions doctors don't seem to understand—chronic fatigue syndrome, sick building syndrome, Gulf War syndrome, and multiple chemical sensitivity syndrome. Alzheimer's disease, Parkinson's disease, arthritis, and hip fractures affect the elderly.

Extensive evidence shows that toxic chemicals can contribute to all of these medical conditions.

And while you may be rightly concerned with air pollution, brace yourself. The air in most homes is two to ten times more polluted than outside air.

WHERE ARE THE TOXINS IN MY HOME?

Consumer products are the leading cause of air pollution in homes. You can make an immediate difference and improve your health and the health of your entire family by learning how to replace toxic products with nontoxic products.

Another major source of indoor air pollution for both homes and businesses is the materials used in interior decorating and construction. Volatile organic compounds in adhesives, paints, and new carpeting, and formaldehyde residues from particle board all emit toxic fumes. By knowing which consumer products and building materials are less toxic and nontoxic, you can learn how to protect yourself and others from a chemical injury.

In addition to indoor air pollution, our food and water can contain residues of toxic chemicals. By learning how to identify the sources of chemical pollution, you will be able to reduce your exposure to these toxins.

The reason most people are confused about toxic chemicals is that the available information is often contradictory. Currently the EPA has 70,000 registered chemicals.[1] No one could learn the names of all the chemicals that have toxic effects, let alone learn information about all of them. You can have a good understanding of the impact of chemicals by focusing on how broad classes of chemicals affect people. This book will teach you about six groups of toxic chemicals:

❖ Pesticides
❖ Petrochemicals
❖ Solvents
❖ Formaldehyde
❖ Heavy metals
❖ Food additives

Here's a brief overview of these six chemical groups.

CLASSES OF NEUROTOXIC CHEMICALS

CLASS OF CHEMICALS: Pesticides

PROPERTIES: Lethal to living organisms

EXAMPLES
Insecticides, herbicides, fungicides

WHERE YOU ARE LIKELY TO ENCOUNTER THEM
❖ Residues are found in food, water, and air supplies
❖ Can concentrate in treated buildings

GENERAL INFORMATION
❖ Derived from chemical warfare
❖ Developed for their neurotoxic properties
❖ Chlorinated hydrocarbon pesticides can remain toxic after twenty years

CLASS OF CHEMICALS: Petrochemicals

PROPERTIES: Hydrocarbon based chemicals

EXAMPLES

Base of many paints, household cleaners, solvents, synthetic fragrances, synthetic materials, synthetic fabrics, food additives, and pesticides

WHERE YOU ARE LIKELY TO ENCOUNTER THEM

Car exhaust fumes, gas appliances, plastics, polyesters, vinyl, fragrances, cosmetics, household cleaners

GENERAL INFORMATION

Many of the chemicals which can be classified as pesticides, solvents, or food additives are also petrochemicals

CLASS OF CHEMICALS: Solvents

PROPERTIES: Dissolve other substances

EXAMPLES

Benzene, toluene, xylene, BTX, styrene, trichloroethylene, ethylbenzene, trimethylbenzene, chloroform

WHERE YOU ARE LIKELY TO ENCOUNTER THEM

❖ Paint thinner, paints, glues, carpet glues, new carpeting, many construction adhesives, octane boosters (BTX, a combination of benzene, toluene, and xylene, can be added to unleaded gasoline), acetone, nail polish remover

❖ Can seep into water supplies from illegal dumps, abandoned dumps, underground storage tanks

GENERAL INFORMATION

❖ Solvent injuries primarily occur in industrial work, and some countries label the phenomenon as solvent syndrome

❖ Elevated levels are found in new or newly remodeled buildings. Solvents are one likely source of sick building syndrome.

❖ Sniffed by inhalant abusers to get high

CLASS OF CHEMICALS: Formaldehyde Based Chemicals

PROPERTIES: Disinfectant, preservative, adhesive component

EXAMPLES
Used as an embalming agent and adhesive

WHERE YOU ARE LIKELY TO ENCOUNTER THEM
Pressboard, mobile homes, carpet glues, new construction, furniture, new carpeting, new clothes, book bindings

GENERAL INFORMATION
❖ Formaldehyde Urea Resin is an inexpensive adhesive
❖ Elevated levels of formaldehyde can be present after construction or remodeling
❖ Another likely source of sick building syndrome

CLASS OF CHEMICALS: Heavy Metals

PROPERTIES: Toxic to the nervous system

EXAMPLES
Lead and mercury

WHERE YOU ARE LIKELY TO ENCOUNTER THEM
Contaminated water supplies (from lead pipes or lead-based solder), leaded paints, residues from leaded gasolines, leaded crystal, silver-mercury fillings in teeth

GENERAL INFORMATION
❖ Lead is a well-known cause of mental retardation in children
❖ Organized studies on mercury toxicity began as early as 1838
❖ Mercury was used in felt hats and led to the phrase "mad as a hatter"

CLASS OF CHEMICALS: Food Additives

PROPERTIES: Used to enhance flavor or color of foods, modify the texture, or as a preservative

EXAMPLES
Excitotoxins (MSG, NutraSweet, Hydrolyzed vegetable protein, and L-cysteine), other artificial flavors, artificial colors, and synthetic preservatives

WHERE YOU ARE LIKELY TO ENCOUNTER THEM
- ❖ NutraSweet is in diet colas and "sugar-free" foods
- ❖ MSG is used in broths, salad dressings, and in many diet and "low fat" foods
- ❖ Artificial colors are in brightly colored cereals, drinks, foods marketed to children
- ❖ All food additives are common in processed, pre-packaged foods

GENERAL INFORMATION
- ❖ Excitotoxins stimulate (or excite) the nerve cells in the brain, sometimes to death
- ❖ There is a long-standing controversy about the effects of synthetic food additives on children

A NONTOXIC LIFESTYLE

Learning to live a nontoxic lifestyle is not like living on some miserable fad diet. It doesn't require you to give up things that are important to you. Rather, it helps you select nontoxic products, such as bug killers, cleaning supplies, detergents, less toxic paints and construction materials, and more wholesome foods that won't cause harm to you or your family. By understanding how toxic chemicals affect human beings in general, you can find out if toxic chemicals might be affecting you. Then you can make good product decisions for yourself and your family.

Have you ever felt irritable or headachy after housecleaning? When Diana used a certain brand of tile cleaner she became nauseated and dizzy for the rest of the afternoon. After she switched to a nontoxic alternative, she was able to clean the tub and stay active the rest of the day.

Janice found that when she quit wearing perfume, her daily headaches went away.

Daniel was about to quit graduate school. He could no longer concentrate and he had frequent migraine headaches. When he quit drinking diet cola, his ability to think returned, the migraines stopped, and he went back to work on his doctorate.

∾

That's what we'll talk about in this book—how toxic chemicals affect the health of real people, not whether they give laboratory rats cancer. What you discover may help you unravel the mystery behind annoying and serious health problems.

You will also learn how toxic chemicals are regulated, so you won't be deceived by labels.

Finally, this book will discuss specific products and nontoxic alternatives. By learning how to replace toxic products with nontoxic products, you can begin to feel better and protect yourself and your family from future health problems.

CHAPTER TWO

Symptoms of a Chemical Injury

Karen couldn't find the words to describe what was happening to her. It was a miserable, tired, depressed, oppressed feeling—like she was walking in a fog with two-ton legs. Her head hurt, she didn't want to eat, she couldn't seem to sleep, and she couldn't seem to wake up. But when she tried to explain it to Dr. Bigley with crisp, businesslike words, all she could say was, "Well, I know something's wrong; I just haven't been feeling well."

Dr. Bigley looked at her sympathetically. She had no fever, her blood tests had come back normal, and she showed no signs of a bacterial or viral infection. He asked about changes in her life and discovered a more promising route of inquiry. She had just been promoted to office manager, and she and her husband were remodeling their home. He asked about the promotion.

"I should like it," Karen said. "I mean, it's work I've done before, but somehow I can't seem to function. I get stressed over every minor detail and can't make decisions. It's not like me. I'm good at deciding—at least I used to be. I made a hundred decisions about the remodeling of our home, but now I just don't seem to care, and I snap at everything. I have headaches and I feel terrible all over. I alternate between feeling stressed—almost hyper—to feeling flat—like I can barely hold up my head."

"Sounds like there's a lot of pressure on you. I mean, at work and at home," Dr. Bigley said. His secretary had just been promoted to office manager and she was not handling the job well. He was beginning to think the promotion had been a mistake. And he remembered how his wife had behaved when they were redecorating their home. They had fought over every detail. He'd considered divorce.

"It shouldn't be this difficult," Karen said. "I've handled much more pressure in the past. Right now I can't seem to handle anything."

"Karen," Dr. Bigley said, "it's okay to admit you can't do everything. I don't think you realize how much stress you're experiencing. It's affecting your health. I'd like to refer you to a psychiatrist I've worked with in the past. He's very good at helping people understand their problems. He can give you something to help you sleep, and maybe he'll refer you for biofeedback to teach you how to reduce stress."

Karen sat quietly on the examining table, her feet dangling over the edge. She wanted to be open to any form of help, but this just didn't seem right. She remembered working with Dr. Terry, a psychologist at the university counseling center, when she was a sophomore in college. Dr. Terry had helped her cope with her parents' divorce. With his help she had identified the conflicts that had always been part of her family, including her father's heavy drinking.

At that time she'd felt angry, sad, and confused, but she hadn't been in as much physical pain as she felt now. Nor had she felt unable to get out of bed. There were a few sleepless nights during that time, but that was because she'd had so much on her mind. This feeling was different. Now, she just couldn't sleep.

Karen also remembered how depression had made her feel. When she and her husband had left her hometown because of his job, she'd felt lonesome and irritable. Her present symptoms were different. Now she was getting lost on the way to familiar places, she couldn't do calculations she'd always done in her head, and she couldn't seem to remember details.

Her promotion should have been easy. She'd already been doing all the work for her former boss; now she was getting credit for it. The only change was moving to the other side of the building. She now had a bigger office, right next to the copy machine. Her first action had been to get the office cleaned and exterminated.

"Doctor, I forgot to mention that I seem to have problems with my memory. I mean, I forget things."

"What's your name?"

"Karen, but I—"

"Where are we?"

"We're in your office. But Doctor, I don't mean big stuff, I mean little things. Like yesterday, I forgot to stop by the cleaners on the way home and—"

She was interrupted by a knock at the door as Dr. Bigley's secretary informed him that his next patient was waiting. He had already spent ten minutes with Karen and prepared to end the appointment.

"I seem to be really uncoordinated, Doctor," Karen said. "I keep dropping things, and I've bumped into the corner of my new desk over and over again. I've actually got a bruise on my hip. You'd think I'd learn the lay of the office."

"Karen, when people are in a state of overload, they can forget to go to the cleaners, and they can bump into furniture when they're too rushed. You need to take a couple of days off to rest, then go more slowly at the new job. Maybe the pressure's too much for you. I also want you to see this psychiatrist. Maybe he can prescribe something for anxiety. I'll tell my secretary to get his number for you."

Karen didn't get a chance to tell Dr. Bigley she'd spent the entire weekend in bed and had been feeling more and more tired for quite a while. Because Dr. Bigley had not been trained to recognize the role toxic chemicals play in illness, he missed the pattern of toxic poisoning Karen described.

COMMON SYMPTOMS OF A CHEMICAL INJURY

This book is about the most dangerous of all chemicals—the ones that poison your brain. These substances are called *neurotoxins,* because they're toxic to your nervous system. The core of the nervous system is the brain, which is the center of our thinking and feeling. The nervous system also regulates every other system in the body. When poisonous substances injure the nervous system, they injure the entire system.

The most common symptoms of neurotoxin poisoning are:

❖ FATIGUE: chronic fatigue, low energy, weakness
❖ MEMORY LOSS: short-term memory loss, poor concentration or comprehension
❖ PERSONALITY CHANGES: irritability, depression, social withdrawal, lack of motivation, lack of ability to think ahead and to plan
❖ HEADACHES: low-grade or severe pain, dizziness, chronic or intermittent pain
❖ SLEEP DISTURBANCES: insomnia, sleeping much more or much less, waking up often
❖ MUSCLE INCOORDINATION: clumsiness, numbness
❖ VISUAL DISTURBANCES: may see "floaters" (spots floating before eyes), may lose peripheral vision
❖ ACHES AND PAINS: joint pain, stomach pain, nausea, general discomfort and achiness
❖ SEXUAL DYSFUNCTION: loss of interest, loss of ability to maintain erection or achieve orgasm, sterility or infertility
❖ RECOGNITION OF LOSS: awareness that there has been a loss of mental functioning; present ability to perform is inferior to past abilities.[1]

These symptoms can be a warning that neurotoxic chemicals may be affecting your health. Let's look at each of them in greater detail.

Fatigue

The most common symptom of neurotoxicity is fatigue, low energy, and weakness. You feel drained, and it's hard even to function.

Neurotoxic fatigue is different from the normal experience of tiredness. Physical exertion and the tiredness it produces is cured by sleep. Neurotoxic fatigue is an unhealthy physical state; sleep doesn't help. Sometimes neurotoxic fatigue can even interfere with the ability to sleep.

A woman, a former sergeant in the army, found herself incapacitated by fatigue after living in a house with a leaky gas furnace. She became so weak that she couldn't button her blouse. This was a woman who used to joke about making up her own bed in the military hospital after delivering her first child. One evening, after the gas exposure, she actually asked her husband to cut her boiled cabbage for her.

Another woman with neurotoxic fatigue said she still went to work, but all she could do when she came home was sleep. She'd lost interest in her friends and social activities. She feared for her future, since she had no family to help her if she could no longer bring home a paycheck. Before she learned how to eliminate neurotoxic chemicals in her home, she felt hopeless about her situation.

The most likely cause of this fatigue is the depletion of one's physical resources by the neurotoxin. I'll explain this process more fully in chapter 6. To summarize, the body exerts energy to eliminate toxins. This process can deplete ATP (cellular energy), enzymes (which cells need to metabolize food sources), and vitamin and mineral reserves. The physical consequence of this excessive cellular exertion may be lethargy and exhaustion.

Neurotoxic fatigue occurs around times of chemical exposure. For example, symptoms may occur after being inside a certain building, when driving in heavy traffic, or after using heavy-duty housecleaning products.

Because each person has a different capacity for physical reserves, some people are affected more quickly than others. People who are in good health should not abuse their bodies and risk future consequences by exposing themselves to neurotoxins.

Memory Loss

Short-term memory loss is a defining characteristic of neurotoxic poisoning. Other early signs of neurotoxicity are absent-mindedness, problems concentrating, confusion, and slow information processing. These cognitive deficits indicate that neurotoxins may be affecting the primary organ of the nervous system, the brain. Mental impairment caused by neurotoxicity can be reversible if there is early intervention.

Another indication of neurotoxicity is when a person begins to perform below his or her normal level. She may suddenly lack the ability to organize simple details and make simple decisions. He may get confused about small things that normally he'd take for granted. While this change in functioning can be difficult to measure on a standardized neuropsychological test, the person affected, and his family, usually know that something is wrong.

Usually, people suffering from neurotoxicity know they're forgetting things (unlike Alzheimer's disease), and it upsets them. Adults will forget about small everyday things and experience difficulty learning new tasks. They may forget the names of friends, get lost on the way to familiar places, forget why they went into a room, or forget words (or syllables of words). If you know someone injured by neurotoxins, you can observe a difference in the way he or she organizes information compared with the way the person used to.

One woman who cleaned houses professionally complained that when she played cards with her children she couldn't remember what had been played from one person's turn to the next. She didn't recover her short-term memory until she quit using toxic cleaning supplies.

Another woman accidentally applied the pesticide chlordane to her clothes. Following the incident, her thinking was so impaired that she couldn't organize information well enough to do household chores or cooking. Four years after the exposure, her thinking was organized enough to cook, but she still had trouble keeping a daily routine.[2]

A surgeon with a toxic exposure was unable to continue his work because he couldn't remember how to perform surgical procedures. He had to go to the library to read about a surgical technique he had invented.

A child who experiences problems with memory and information processing will have difficulty learning new material in a classroom setting, which could look like a learning disability. Unlike an adult, a child, especially a very young child, cannot report that her thinking processes have changed, because she has no point of reference. The people around her may not realize that her ability to remember and process information has decreased. It's more obvious if an older child suddenly begins to have problems learning. In both cases, consider the possibility of neurotoxic poisoning.

While psychological stress or depression can impact memory by interfering with concentration, stress and depression follow a different pattern than neurotoxicity. Most people know when they've undergone a trauma or when they're distracted. It's the inability to remember daily routine things, even when concentrating, that's more typical of chemical injuries. If an office is renovated and the staff find they are tired, forgetful, and prone to making errors in their work, they may be showing signs of neurotoxicity.

Personality Changes

When neurotoxic chemicals alter brain functioning, they can also alter emotional experiences. People who are exposed to neurotoxins may become irritable, angry, depressed, socially withdrawn, unmotivated, and unable to think ahead or to plan ahead.

When someone who is not normally angry or depressed takes on these characteristics, it may indicate a neurotoxic exposure. Another indication would be if these symptoms appear when the person is working at a certain location or uses a certain product.

Neurotoxic chemicals are capable of changing all mental processes, including emotions and personality traits, by altering brain functioning. Many substances are intentionally used for this purpose. Inhalants, such as glues and paints (which are solvents), are abused specifically for their mind-altering properties. Illegal drugs and alcohol are used to change mood and perception. Psychiatric medications are prescribed to change brain chemistry. Other prescribed drugs can also temporarily affect emotions or personality.

When a person experiences emotion, the brain releases neuropeptides—amino acid chains—to communicate throughout the nervous system and the rest of the body. When you feel angry, neuropeptides prepare your body for action. Blood flow, for example, increases in the muscles and the brain to prepare you for fight or flight. If the neuropeptides are triggered by something else, such as a neurotoxic chemical, the body's response is the same. The body cannot discern a false alarm. As the saying goes, you get "all stressed up and no one to choke."

Toxins can conjure up anger or depression, just as chemicals like alcohol or heroin trigger certain emotional experiences. With a chemical exposure, however, the person affected is unlikely to know what's happening to her or what's causing her emotion.

In one Texas automobile manufacturing plant, physical fights were breaking out every Friday afternoon in the paint department. An astute human resources member checked the filtration system and found it needed repair. When the week-long accumulation of paint fumes ended, the fights ended.

Altered mental and emotional functioning can even lead to life-threatening situations. In an investigation of one incident in which a crop-duster pilot crashed into power lines, the pilot reported that his judgment was so impaired after exposure to his toxic load of pesticides that even though he knew he was about to crash, he didn't care.[3]

A more common situation in daily life is interacting with others. When a person's thinking and feeling is altered by toxins, there can be an increase in conflicts, which can have a devastating effect on marriage and family life.

Headaches

Severe and persistent headaches and dizziness are a common symptom of neurotoxicity. Of course, headaches and dizziness are also a common symptom of other injuries, diseases, or stresses. If your headaches are caused by a toxic exposure, they will stop after you end your exposure to the toxin.

One young school teacher suffered from migraine headaches. She gave up teaching and began a part-time job because she thought the headaches were related to stress. One day she learned about neurotoxins in housecleaning products. When she switched to nontoxic products, the headaches stopped. She was able to return to teaching without further problems.

Another woman quit wearing perfume when she found that a friend had a serious sensitivity to fragrance. About a month later she realized she hadn't experienced her familiar headaches for a month. She wondered if there was a connection, and she put on some of her perfume. The headaches returned.

A man found that his headaches were increasing in severity and intensity. His doctor could find no cause, and the painkillers he prescribed were becoming less and less effective. A coworker finally convinced the man his headaches might be caused by NutraSweet. The man was ready to try anything, so he stopped drinking diet colas. The headaches stopped. His experience is not unusual; many people find that NutraSweet causes headaches.[4]

Since the brain is the organ under attack from neurotoxins, it makes sense that neurotoxins cause headaches. The real cause of headaches, however, is not straightforward, because brain cells do not have pain receptors.

If you've seen brain surgery on TV, you know they do not use anesthesia, because the actual brain cells do not register pain. Scientists don't know exactly what causes headaches. One theory is that headaches are the result of pain receptors in the brain's blood vessels.[5] If there is inflammation and swelling in the brain, it could press on the blood vessels and cause the pain sensation.

Because pain receptors warn us if there's an injury to our bodies, the fact that brain cells do not have pain receptors is important in understanding how chemical injuries can occur. The lack of a warning system is what makes the brain so vulnerable to slow, chronic injury. The slow degeneration of brain cells is called "silent" brain damage, because a person may not know anything is wrong until there is severe impairment.

If you don't have symptoms of neurotoxicity, you can't assume that neurotoxic chemicals aren't affecting you. The brain doesn't hurt like other organs of the body. Conditions such as Alzheimer's disease or Parkinson's disease can appear after years of exposure with no early warning symptoms.

Sleep Disturbances

Insomnia is a common symptom in people affected by neurotoxins. Many people with neurotoxic injuries become night owls, unable to fall asleep at night and unable to rouse from sleep in the morning. They may wake frequently in the night and have bad dreams. Their disturbed sleep increases their fatigue. Some people find they need more sleep after a chemical injury. Often when people with neurotoxic poisoning wake up in the morning, they wake up in pain.

Sleep disturbances can be an indication of depression, but depression tends to follow a different pattern. Typically, someone with clinical depression is able to fall asleep at night but wakes up in the early morning hours and can't return to sleep.

The typical sleep pattern from neurotoxicity is difficulty going to sleep at night and difficulty waking in the morning. Some people with neurotoxic injuries are unable to function in the morning due to the altered sleep pattern and morning pain.

Serotonin is a chemical the brain uses to regulate the sleep-wake cycle, and it's likely that a serotonin imbalance causes sleep problems. We'll learn about the role of important brain chemicals like serotonin in chapter 3.

Incidentally, aspartame, found in NutraSweet, can alter serotonin levels,[6] so it would be important for people with insomnia to avoid this artificial sweetener.

Muscle Incoordination

Since the nervous system controls muscle movement and sensations, damage to the nervous system can alter muscular functioning. Neurotoxic poisoning can show itself in muscle incoordination, muscle weakness, and numbness.

The most common cause of neurotoxicity in industrial settings is solvent exposures, which often cause muscle numbness and weakness.

Several workers in one manufacturing plant were poisoned by the solvent methyl n-butyl. They experienced weakness in the hands and feet and difficulty grasping heavy objects. They reported they could barely turn a key, click a cigarette lighter, or use a screwdriver. Several of the men had trouble walking.[7]

When weakness, incoordination, or numbness occur in an industrial setting, there is increased risk of accidents. A worker who is losing coordination can be hurt by heavy machinery or make an error that injures someone else. It's not known how often neurotoxicity plays a role in accidents, but neurotoxic symptoms such as impaired manual dexterity, visual perception, and short-term memory all increase the risk. Accidents are one of the hidden costs of neurotoxic chemicals.[8]

The effect of low-level poisoning may be subtle. A person can compensate for some loss of coordination by concentrating on each movement. But when someone consistently drops dishes, gets bruised from walking into furniture, or begins to lose coordination in a favorite sport, it's time to consider a neurotoxic injury. A loss of muscular control is most obvious in complex muscle movements, such as playing a musical instrument, operating precision tools, or typing.

Subtle forms of incoordination take a toll. One woman mourned that in the course of her first year of marriage she had dropped and broken all of her glass wedding presents. A teenage musician had to drop out of a musical competition because he was losing finger coordination, despite practicing two hours a day. A secretary explained that she only wore flat shoes because she never knew when she would lose her balance and didn't want to twist an ankle.

Visual Disturbances

Some people injured by neurotoxic chemicals report blurred vision, loss of peripheral vision (tunnel vision), the presence of "floaters" (black spots), the need for more light to see, or that too much light bothers their eyes. Some people even report that their vision prescriptions changed after a chemical exposure.

One crop-duster pilot who was accidentally exposed to his load of pesticides reported blurred vision and difficulty finding the landing field. Another pilot reported "stovepipe vision" (tunnel vision), which initially prevented him from landing.[9]

A person's visual system is physically located in the brain. When the eye sees an image, the optic nerve carries signals from the eyes to the occipital lobe of the brain, which interprets these signals. Any pressure to the optic nerve can cause distortions in vision.

Both MSG and NutraSweet have the potential to cause visual problems. As early as 1957, scientists found that MSG destroyed the nerve cells in the inner layer of the retina in mice.[10] Symptoms of blurred vision, bright flashes of light, tunnel vision, and blindness have been attributed to NutraSweet.[11] Several pilots have lost their medical certification (they can no longer fly) due to visual problems or seizures which they attribute to NutraSweet.[12]

Aches and Pains

Sometimes people who are exposed to neurotoxins report flu-like symptoms. Other common complaints include general achiness, joint pain, nausea, or stomach pain.

To understand pain caused by neurotoxicity, it's important to understand how the body perceives any type of pain.

We experience pain as a result of brain activity. The brain gives and receives messages through the nervous system. If you break your leg, the nervous system relays a signal from the leg to the brain. Your brain then creates the sensation of pain, and that pain is experienced in the leg. This entire process occurs almost instantaneously. The reason drugs like morphine effectively block pain is not because they help your leg but because they change your brain's perception of pain.

Since the brain is the source of all pain experiences, it makes sense that a chemical which alters brain functioning could alter the perception of pain. A person could experience "phantom" pain—a message of pain in a part of the body that isn't injured or a pain whose location they can't describe. They may feel pain when no signal has been sent to the brain from the body, or they may feel exaggerated pain.

In cases of neurotoxic poisoning, a person can experience pain that is entirely within the brain, pain that is due to actual cell damage at the source of the pain, or pain for both reasons.

Nausea is controlled by a part of the brain called the thalamus. If someone with neurotoxic overexposure is feeling nauseated, it could indicate digestive difficulties, a problem in the thalamus in the brain, or both conditions.

Sexual Dysfunction
The most frequent type of sexual dysfunction in men with neurotoxic poisoning is difficulty maintaining an erection. Both men and women can experience a loss of sexual interest, due to fatigue and irritability.[13] Researchers probably are underestimating the impact of neurotoxins on sexual functioning, because many people do not admit to sexual problems.

In one case, National Institute of Occupational Safety and Health (NIOSH) investigators accidentally learned about sexual dysfunctions while interviewing workers suffering from neurotoxic poisoning in a plant that synthesized polyurethane foam for seat cushions. The men reported tingling in their hands and feet and problems with urination. While investigating the bladder complaints, investigators also learned the men were unable to have an erection.[14]

Sterility can be another consequence of neurotoxicity. Many toxic substances are known to reduce sperm density. As the production of neurotoxic chemicals increases, the average sperm density in the population at large is decreasing.[15]

Because of the close interconnection between the nervous system and the endocrine (hormonal) system, endocrine function is vulnerable to neurotoxins. Some toxins, particularly organophosphate pesticides and PCBs, have an estrogenlike activity. This means a toxin could trigger a response in the body that is normally triggered by estrogen.

These estrogen imitators seem to be particularly dangerous to women and are thought to contribute to breast cancer, endometriosis, premenstrual syndrome (PMS), thyroid disorders, and infertility. Some researchers are examining the connection between these toxins and early puberty in girls.[16]

Recognition of Loss

People who have been injured by neurotoxins know *something* is wrong. They may or may not know if they were exposed to a neurotoxic chemical, but they know they're not the same. They lack energy they used to have; they feel bad; they forget things they never used to forget; their performance is down; their coordination has deteriorated; their motivation and interest are gone.

In short, they're different.

In some cases, neurotoxicity begins slowly, with vague symptoms of low energy, clumsiness, memory loss, and discomfort. It can be hard for someone to verbalize what's happening. In other cases, neurotoxicity shows up immediately on the heels of an exposure to a specific known toxin. In either case, people with neurotoxic injuries know and can report that something has changed, and they don't feel normal.

When people with neurotoxic injuries are tested on measures of intelligence, they tend to do better on tests that measure past learning rather than present abilities. That's because long-term memory can stay intact, while short-term memory is severely impaired.

Sometimes patients with excellent academic backgrounds cannot perform simple tasks after a neurotoxic injury. For example, a student in a calculus course made errors in single-digit addition while understanding complex mathematical proofs. An athletic person may find he's unable to coordinate movements that have always come naturally.

The loss of an ability can be a significant indicator of a pathological process in the brain. This important clue to neurotoxicity can be overlooked by professional health-care providers because it's difficult to measure objectively. After all, just because someone says he used to have a skill doesn't mean he did. Astute health professionals will want to know about these changes and will want to hear from family members about the changes they've observed. These losses in functioning provide a measure of the injury and of recovery.

HEEDING EARLY WARNING SIGNS

Symptoms such as memory loss, confusion, fatigue, and personality changes should be taken seriously. They may be warning signs of neurotoxic poisoning. As one behavioral toxicologist described it, "Many poisonings, before they bloom into overt clinical signs, may be heralded by vague, subjective, nonspecific psychological complaints."[17]

If a person heeds early warning signs, toxicity can be reversed and healthy functioning resumed. When an injury to the brain has progressed to the point of Alzheimer's disease or Parkinson's disease, the tissue damage is so severe that little can be done to reverse it.

୦୰

Now that you know the ten most commonly reported symptoms of neurotoxicity, you may want to read the beginning of this chapter again to see if you recognize a pattern for yourself in the symptoms Karen reported to her doctor. Because she and her doctor were uninformed about neurotoxicity, they couldn't see the pattern of symptoms or the sources of her neurotoxic exposures. Karen's real problems went undetected and untreated.

CHAPTER THREE

How Chemicals Affect Your Nervous System

If you want to understand how neurotoxic chemicals injure the body, you need to understand how the nervous system works.

When you see the prefix *neuro-*, it refers to nerve cells or the nervous system. A neuron is a nerve cell, neuronal communication is communication between nerve cells, and neurology is the medical study of the nervous system.

You may be tempted right now to skip the next several chapters and jump to the practical chapters on how to live a nontoxic lifestyle. I urge you to read the next five chapters carefully. In order to protect yourself from chemical injuries, you need to understand why your body is vulnerable to neurotoxic poisoning. The more you know about how your body works, the better equipped you will be to prevent and treat neurological damage.

THE NERVOUS SYSTEM

When we study a road map, we see that it differentiates between highways and surface streets, even though both roads contribute to one objective. In a similar way, when doctors and scientists study the nervous system, they divide it into sections for the sake of conve-

32

nience. These divisions in the nervous system do not actually exist, because all the parts of the nervous system work together.

The nervous system can be divided by location or function. The first major division is between the central nervous system and the peripheral nervous system (figure 3.1).

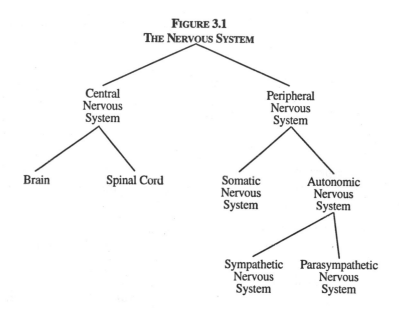

FIGURE 3.1
THE NERVOUS SYSTEM

The Central Nervous System
The central nervous system refers to the brain and the spinal cord, which are so important to the body that they're encased in bone. This is the maximum protection the body can provide.

The Brain
We take for granted many of the brain's numerous functions. You probably know that your brain is the center of learning, communicating, perceiving experiences, remembering past events, and feeling emotions. But you may not know that your brain helps regulate the functions of life, such as breathing and blood circulation, hunger, thirst, temperature, and muscle movements. Chemicals that are toxic to the nervous system endanger the functioning of the entire body.

Serious injury to the brain can end the ability to think, speak, and control movements, or even end life.

The Spinal Cord

The spinal cord is the major pathway for the nerves between the brain and all the muscles and organs in the body. Your spine protects the nerve pathways so the brain can control movement and receive input from the body. Serious injury to the spinal cord can result in paralysis.

The Peripheral Nervous System

The peripheral nervous system is located outside, or on the periphery, of the central nervous system. It functions as the body's communication system, and its importance to life and to functioning cannot be overestimated.

The peripheral nervous system can be divided into two parts, based on function: the somatic and the autonomic nervous systems.

The Somatic Nervous System

Somatic is derived from the Greek word *soma,* which means "the body." The somatic nervous system controls voluntary muscle movements and relays sensations back to the brain. The nerves that carry information from the brain to the muscles relay information about contracting or releasing. The nerves that carry information from the muscles to the brain communicate experiences of pain, temperature, pressure, and touch.

When you walk across a room, your somatic nervous system relays information from your brain to move the muscles of your legs and feet. If you stub your toe on the coffee table, the somatic nervous system relays that message of pain back to your brain. The somatic nervous system also relays information to your vocal cords so that you can yell "OWWW!" (or anything else).

The Autonomic Nervous System

The autonomic nervous system is the communication system for the organs. Think of it as regulating the automatic functions of the body—the heart and the lungs, digestion, the sexual response, and the stress (adrenal) response. This system controls muscles you don't think about—such as those that surround your blood vessels and the bronchia in your lungs. The autonomic nervous system has gotten more press lately because of interest in stress and the role it plays in promoting disease.

The autonomic nervous system contains two subsystems that are important in both crisis situations and restful times. One subsystem, the sympathetic nervous system, responds to emergencies and crises. In situations of fear or anger, your body prepares for action. The sympathetic nervous system directs blood into the heart, lungs, and large muscles so that you can move. You may remember how you felt the last time you had stage fright—pounding heart, fast breathing, dry mouth, feelings of apprehension. Your sympathetic nervous system was getting your body ready to fight your best or to run away.

The other subsystem—the parasympathetic nervous system—regulates quiet, vegetative functioning, such as rest and digestion. The heart beats at a slower pace when the parasympathetic system is in control. You may notice that your hands are warmer when you're calm and relaxed; this is because the parasympathetic nervous system reduces the blood flow to your heart, lungs, and large muscles after the crisis is over, and it increases circulation in your hands, digestive system, and other organs. Mood rings and stress monitors work by measuring the temperature in your hand, which roughly estimates parasympathetic activity.

Usually, either the sympathetic or the parasympathetic system is in operation. But sometimes both systems work together, as in sexual functioning.

To summarize, the nervous system is subdivided because it is so versatile and performs so many functions. Your nervous system regulates the functioning of every muscle and organ in your body. For any action or thought to occur, a nerve cell somewhere has to relay a message.

NEURONS AND NEUROTRANSMITTERS

The functioning of the entire nervous system is based on a series of communications sent from one nerve cell to another. Neurons (nerve cells) have a chain of communication in which one neuron communicates to the next one, until the last neuron in the chain communicates directly to a target muscle or a target organ.

The communication between nerve cells is an amazing process. In figure 3.2 you can see a simple drawing of two nerve cells. The body of a neuron is similar to other cells in the body but has a projection, called an axon, that extends to the next neuron. Nerve cells communicate both through the axon and through dendrites (the smaller projections). Axons vary in length. In the brain, where many neurons are right next to each other, the axons are short. The axons that extend all the way down to your feet are long. At the end of the axon, a chemical is released which transmits the message of the neuron. This substance is called a neurotransmitter. The next neuron in the chain is designed to receive the neurotransmitter.

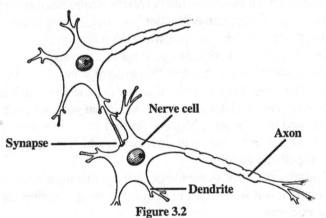

Figure 3.2

Reprinted from *Mayo Clinic Family Health Book*, 1990, William Morrow and Company, New York. With permission of Mayo Foundation for Medical Education and Research, and William Morrow and Company, Inc., Publisher, New York.

There are many different neurotransmitters; currently we know of about fifty. Some of the best known and understood neurotransmitters are dopamine, epinephrine, norepinephrine, serotonin, and acetylcholine. Some amino acids act as neurotransmitters, including glutamate, aspartate, and glycine.[1]

Neurotransmitters are the substance of communication in the nervous system and are critical to human functioning. Some real-life examples may help you grasp just how important they are by showing what happens when they're out of balance.

When a person's nervous system is low on the neurotransmitter dopamine, he loses muscular control. Parkinson's disease is a condition in which a person increasingly loses muscular control. One of the treatments for Parkinson's disease is a drug called L-Dopa, which increases the body's ability to produce dopamine.

On the other hand, an excess of dopamine can cause hallucinations. It's believed that people who suffer from schizophrenia have an excess of dopamine, because the most effective medications for schizophrenia are ones that reduce the amount of dopamine in the nervous system.

When it comes to neurotransmitters, too much of a good thing is just too much. If patients with Parkinson's take enough medication to create an excess of dopamine, they can experience hallucinations. On the other hand, patients who are being treated for schizophrenia are at risk of developing Parkinson's symptoms — loss of muscular control — when they take an excess of dopamine-reducing medications.

The brain maintains a delicate balance with a specific range for each neurotransmitter. Too much or too little of the message-bearing chemicals can be devastating.

The drug L-Dopa was used by the doctor in the movie *Awakenings,* starring Robin Williams and Robert DeNiro. If you saw this movie, you will probably never forget how important the right amount of dopamine is for human functioning.

Another crucial neurotransmitter is acetylcholine (pronounced a-seat-ill-ko-leen). Acetylcholine is used every time you move a muscle in your body, and not just the skeletal muscles you typically think about. Acetylcholine also works to facilitate the smooth muscles in organs such as the heart, lungs, and digestive tract. Our bodies have a built-in "safety factor" to make sure these muscles work: The neurons release three to four times the needed amount of acetylcholine to make sure the muscle fibers are stimulated at the right time.[2]

Acetylcholine has other functions in the body that we don't understand as well. Apparently, acetylcholine plays some role in the immune system.[3] Acetylcholine also plays an important role in memory. A deficiency of acetylcholine has been associated with Alzheimer's disease.[4]

Acetylcholine has to be removed from the gap between neurons each time it is released because the neuron can't transmit the next message until it's removed. An enzyme called acetylcholinesterase exists for this very purpose. (You can think of acetylcholines*terase* as erasing acetylcholine.)

Your very life depends on the process of releasing and removing neurotransmitters. When scientists wanted to invent deadly weapons for war, they developed a toxic substance—nerve gas—that would destroy the enzyme acetylcholinesterase. Without the enzyme, too much acetylcholine builds up in the gaps between the neurons and causes the receiving muscles and organs to work very hard and fast until they collapse from exhaustion. The heart beats wildly at first, but then it stops beating altogether.

In war, American soldiers carry a drug—atropine—to counteract the effects of nerve gas. Besides treating people exposed to chemical warfare, atropine has only one other use—to treat people exposed to chemical pesticides.

Organophosphate pesticides and carbamate pesticides kill by destroying acetylcholinesterase. It's not a coincidence that these pesticides act like chemical weapons. They are the direct descendants of chemical warfare.

∽

Once you understand how the nervous system regulates and controls the functioning of the body, you can understand how an injury to the nervous system—whose symptoms were described in chapter 2—can result in so many damaging consequences.

In the next chapter, we'll talk about how the nervous system regulates five critical systems in your body and how neurotoxins can cause or contribute to diseases and syndromes in these systems.

CHAPTER FOUR

NEUROTOXINS AND THE DISEASE PROCESS

THE NERVOUS SYSTEM

The human brain is amazing in its capabilities. It's also vulnerable because it lacks pain receptors. Even while the brain is being injured, it continues to operate and compensate for the injury, unless the destruction becomes too widespread.

If you don't know that your brain is being injured, you'll probably continue exposing yourself to the cause of the injury. By the time you notice a loss of functioning, the injury can be quite extensive. In some cases, a disease process is not detected until the damage is beyond repair.

All brain functions are vulnerable to neurotoxins, because these substances are poisonous to the brain cells. Neurotoxic poisoning causes neurological injuries that can cause or contribute to conditions such as Alzheimer's disease and other dementias, Parkinson's disease, and amyotrophic lateral sclerosis (ALS, or Lou Gehrig's disease). These are neurodegenerative diseases, which means they follow a slow course of brain deterioration. These dreaded conditions are called "diseases" because of the destruction they cause to the lives of people, not because they are caused by germs.

Alzheimer's Disease and Other Dementia

Dementia is the generalized brain deterioration we associate with old age, which causes memory loss and confusion.

Dementia can result from stroke, injury, disease, or deterioration of the brain. Brain cells are particularly vulnerable to an injury because they do not regenerate. Once a neuron is destroyed, it's gone forever. Although we have billions of neurons, the erosion of neurons over a lifetime can eventually cause so much destruction that a person can't continue to function normally.

Increasingly, researchers in the field of aging are looking at the role neurotoxins play in dementia.[1] For example, the neurons destroyed in Alzheimer's disease are those that produce acetylcholine.[2] As we found in chapter 3, most pesticides alter the acetylcholine cycle. It's not known how many cases of Alzheimer's disease are caused by neurotoxicity or in how many cases neurotoxicity contributes by making a person more vulnerable to factors that could cause Alzheimer's disease.[3]

Parkinson's Disease

Parkinson's disease is another debilitating neurodegenerative condition in which early symptoms indicate that severe damage has occurred. By the time a person knows something is wrong, there is already extensive damage to a structure in the brain known as the *substantia nigra*. The *substantia nigra* is part of the nigrostriatal system in the brain, which controls movement. This structure uses the neurotransmitter dopamine to communicate.

The toxic link became apparent in the 1980s when a young man developed full-blown Parkinson's disease overnight. Normally, Parkinson's disease is a slow, degenerative process seen in older adults. This young man had taken MPTP—a synthetic version of heroin. This shocking case prompted studies between neurotoxic chemical exposures and the onset of Parkinson's disease.

Some cases of Parkinson's disease or a similar condition have been linked to carbon monoxide, carbon disulfide, mercury, and pesticide exposures.[4] Neurotoxic exposures can work slowly compared to the "designer drug" MPTP, but the end result may be the same.

Evidence that people from rural communities are more likely to get Parkinson's disease has led to research on the role of neurotoxic pesticides as the cause or as a contributing factor to this condition. In agricultural areas, entire communities are exposed to neurotoxic pesticides that seep into ground water supplies. One study found that the rates of Parkinson's disease varied in six different water districts in Quebec, Canada, based on pesticide sales within the district. The districts that bought more pesticides had more cases of Parkinson's disease.[5] Another study in Quebec found that districts using more pesticides had more cases of "region specific" Parkinson's disease.[6]

ALS (Lou Gehrig's Disease)

Another frightening neurodegenerative disease is amyotrophic lateral sclerosis (ALS), more commonly known as Lou Gehrig's disease. In ALS, there is a slow deterioration of the nerve cells in the brain and spinal cord that control muscle movement. Muscles depend on the nerve cells to stimulate movement. As one set of nerve cells after another deteriorates, the muscle fibers become useless and waste away. This disease is a slow, creeping form of paralysis.

The causes of this disease are unknown. Neurotoxic chemicals, particularly the heavy metals, are one suspect among many.

Neurotoxic chemicals could be a culprit in a large proportion of neurodegenerative diseases. In some cases, neurotoxins are the sole cause of the neurodegenerative process, and in other cases, neurotoxins play a contributing role.

Mental Illness

Sometimes people who are injured by neurotoxins manifest psychotic symptoms. You may have heard the expression, "Mad as a hatter." Insanity was an occupational hazard for hatmakers who used mercury to make felt hats. Neurotoxins can cause hallucinations, an impaired ability to communicate, and an impaired ability to function in society.[7]

A person who's been poisoned by neurotoxins can have symptoms similar to depression, such as fatigue, irritability, and sleep disturbances. However, neurotoxicity is different from clinical depression. A significant difference is that neurotoxicity causes short-term memory loss. Another difference is that people suffering from neurotoxicity do not show the distortions in thinking that define clinical depression—

feelings of worthlessness, guilt, and hopelessness.[8] This isn't to say that people who've been poisoned by neurotoxins do not get depressed. They get depressed because they're fatigued, not fatigued because they're depressed.

Seizures

A seizure, also called a convulsion, occurs when the normal electrical discharges in the brain get disorganized. Abnormal electrical activity in the brain causes an uncontrolled episode of alternating muscle contraction and relaxation and can be caused by various conditions such as epilepsy, a high fever, kidney failure, or certain drugs and poisons[9]—including an acute neurotoxic exposure.[10]

THE ENDOCRINE SYSTEM

The endocrine system is made up of glands that release chemical messengers called hormones. Hormones circulate throughout the body carrying messages to other organs. The endocrine system includes the pituitary gland (part of the brain), the thyroid gland (located in the neck), the pancreas, the adrenal gland, and reproductive organs (ovaries and testes). These glands communicate with one another and regulate the body by circulating hormones in the bloodstream.

Most people are familiar with the hormones released by the ovaries and testes—estrogen, progesterone, and testosterone. You've probably also heard of insulin, which is the hormone produced by the pancreas. Your pituitary gland released growth hormone when you were a child, and it continues to release an antidiuretic hormone, called vasopressin, which regulates the water content of your body. Your thyroid gland releases several hormones, including thyroxine, an important regulatory hormone that increases the rate of cell metabolism. In times of excitement or crisis, your adrenal gland releases adrenalin.

Like the nervous system, the endocrine system is a regulatory system. The endocrine system is so closely connected to the nervous system that doctors refer to their interconnection as the "neuroendocrine axis." In fact, your adrenal gland is a hybrid between the two systems. Technically it's an endocrine gland, but the adrenalin it releases is also called epinephrine, which is a neurotransmitter. The endocrine system is responsive to both hormonal messages and neurotransmitter messages. If either set of messages gets altered, the endocrine system is affected. Changes in the amount of hormones released can dramatically affect your health and well-being.

Endocrine dysfunctions that may be linked to neurotoxicity include thyroid disorders (particularly hypothyroidism), premenstrual syndrome (PMS), and endometriosis.[11] Hypothyroidism, which means that the thyroid is underactive, may make a person more susceptible to future exposures to neurotoxins. Endometriosis has recently been linked to dioxin (a toxic byproduct of herbicide), waste water from paper and pulp companies, and incineration. The numerous toxins in cigarette smoke increase the chances of reduced fertility, pregnancy complications, premature birth, low birth weight, stillbirth, and infant mortality.[12]

The endocrine system is vulnerable to neurotoxins in three ways. First, an alteration in the nervous system has the potential to affect the endocrine system.

Second, neurotoxins can accumulate in the endocrine organs. When silver-mercury dental amalgams were placed in the mouth of a female sheep, the mercury accumulated in the pituitary, thyroid, adrenal, pancreas, and ovary.[13]

Third, neurotoxins can affect the endocrine system by triggering hormonal responses. For example, certain toxins, called xenoestrogens (pronounced *zee-no-estrogens*), have an estrogenlike activity. These toxins fool the body into responding to them as if they were estrogen and can trigger estrogen responses at the wrong time, with damaging results. Researchers are examining the role of xenoestrogens in breast cancer, reproductive disorders, and endometriosis. It's possible that xenoestrogens are linked to girls reaching puberty at younger ages. Xenoestrogen chemicals include organophosphate pesticides and PCBs.[14]

THE IMMUNE SYSTEM

Your immune system activates and regulates your body's defenses against disease. It defends you against cancer and viral, fungal, and bacterial infections by labeling the cells of your body "self," and everything else as "non-self." The most famous immunological disease is Acquired Immune Deficiency Syndrome (AIDS), which is believed to be caused by the HIV virus.

The field of psychoneuroimmunology studies how the brain, the neuroendocrine system, and the immune system influence one another.[15] Scientists are only beginning to understand the close interconnection between the nervous system and the immune system, but research has discovered that nerve cells release neurotransmitters directly into immune system organs.[16] It appears that these systems use neurotransmitters, neurohormones, and neuropeptides to communicate information to one another, especially when the immune system is actively fighting off a disease.[17]

It's been shown in animal studies that injuring or removing parts of the brain results in significant decreases in immune system function.[18] This indicates that a brain injury—caused by chemicals or something else—may have an effect on immune system function.

Toxic chemicals have the potential to alter immune function indirectly by damaging the nervous system or directly by injuring the cells of the immune system.

The field of immunotoxicology studies the effects of toxic chemicals and drugs on the immune system.[19] An example of one neurotoxin that can alter immune function is the pesticide chlordane, which is used to kill termites. People accidentally exposed to chlordane were found to have altered immune function, including immune deficiency, dysregulation of both T and B cells, and evidence of early signs of autoimmunity.[20] Mercury is another neurotoxin with the potential to precipitate autoimmunity.[21]

Injury to your immune system could result in "catching" every bug that goes around or the inability to fight off a virus; it could increase your risk for cancer, or your body could activate its attack system at the wrong time and against the wrong thing.

Allergies flare up when the immune system is triggered by a substance that is typically benign. When someone has an autoimmune disorder, her immune cells attack the cells of her own body. Rheumatoid arthritis, lupus, multiple sclerosis, and myasthenia gravis are autoimmune disorders. Some thyroid disorders result from an autoimmune response. Incidentally, excess fluoride can lead to skeletal fluorosis, which is likely to be misdiagnosed as arthritis because the symptoms are similar.

The causes of autoimmune disease are poorly understood, but neurotoxic chemicals have the potential to contribute to these conditions in the following ways.

First, neurotoxins could interfere with neuroimmune communication.

Second, neurotoxins could damage developing immune cells. Immune cells develop in bone marrow, and neurotoxins stored in bone marrow would have access to them. This could result in defective immune cells.

Third, neurotoxins could cause cells to mutate (which is how they're thought to cause cancer). The immune system should attack a mutated cell, which is how it prevents cancer.

Normally, the immune system does not attack healthy "self cells" because they have an identification code. When a cell is mutated, its identification code reflects the change. If the change is slight, the attack on the slightly changed cells could trigger an attack on healthy cells.

Once an attack on "self" begins, it can self-perpetuate. The immune system is designed to destroy foreign organisms labeled "non-self." If your own body is mislabeled as "non-self," it will be under destructive attack by the system that was designed to protect it.

Although autoimmune diseases are not fully understood, it is clear that women are more prone to them than men. In the case of lupus, the ratio is about nine women for every man.[22] It is thought that estrogen plays some role in making women more vulnerable to autoimmune diseases. Both estrogen and testosterone have been shown to influence the immune response.[23] It is possible that the xenoestrogens (the hormone impostors) have an estrogenlike effect on the immune system. These deceptive neurotoxins may have the potential to alter immune functioning.

The functioning of the immune system is very complex. Any interference with this system can lead to health problems. For instance, a weakened immune system can leave a person vulnerable to bacterial, viral, and yeast infections; cancer can develop when the immune system is unable to destroy mutated cells; and if the immune system mislabels the cells of the body, it causes an autoimmune disease.

THE CARDIOVASCULAR SYSTEM

The nervous system has direct physical control over the cardiovascular system—the heart, lungs, and blood vessels—through neural impulses. Since these smooth muscles are involuntary muscles—they work whether we think about them or not—the nervous system constantly regulates them to maintain functioning.

When it's cold outside, your hands and feet get cold first. This happens when sensory nerve cells in your skin signal to your brain that it's cold. Your brain sends signals through the autonomic nervous system to the smooth muscles that surround the blood vessels in your hands and feet. This signal causes your blood vessels to constrict, reducing the blood flow in your hands and feet, so that less blood circulates near the skin where it can be cooled by the outside temperature. This allows your body to maintain a warm temperature and protect your life.

When it's hot outside, your nervous system will expand the size of the blood vessels near the skin so that more blood can come to the surface to be cooled.

When you're in a dangerous situation, your nervous system increases blood flow to vital organs to prepare you for action.

Neurotoxic chemicals can directly affect the cardiovascular system. Inhaled cigarette smoke is a known risk factor in heart disease, and organophosphate pesticides are known to cause high blood pressure. When the vessels constrict, the heart must pump harder at each stroke to move the blood throughout the body. This puts constant increased pressure on the heart and increases the risk of heart attack and stroke.

No one knows how large a role neurotoxins play in causing or contributing to high blood pressure and heart disease, but avoiding cigarette smoke, neurotoxic pesticides, and other neurotoxins are wise precautions for protecting your heart.

THE GASTROINTESTINAL SYSTEM

The nervous system also controls the smooth muscles involved in digestion. The neurotransmitters acetylcholine, gastrin-releasing peptide (GRP), and histamine are all important in digestion.[24] The parasympathetic nervous system regulates this process. Damage to the nervous system could interfere with its regulation of the gastrointestinal system.

The gastrointestinal system also has contact with neurotoxins in food, water, or medicines. When neurotoxins are ingested, the cells of the digestive system have to divert their function from the metabolism of nutrients to the biotransformation and detoxification of neurotoxins (see chapter 6). During digestion, these substances have direct contact with the stomach and intestines.

Some of the conditions associated with neurotoxic chemical injuries to this system include digestive problems, food intolerance, food allergies, and irritable bowel syndrome.[25]

SYNDROMES CAUSED BY NEUROTOXICITY

In recent years, there have been increasing reports of chemical injury syndromes. Solvent syndrome, sick building syndrome, multiple chemical sensitivity syndrome, and Gulf War syndrome are all controversial diagnoses that follow a similar pattern. These syndromes and others are characterized by neurotoxic symptoms often accompanied by endocrine, immune, cardiovascular, or gastrointestinal disorders.

Solvent syndrome, sick building syndrome, and Gulf War syndrome are all named for the alleged source of the toxic exposure. In the Gulf War, there was a continuous exposure to petrochemicals due to burning oil wells. If chemical weapons were used, they would be likely to cause a neurotoxic injury similar to organophosphate pesticide poisoning.

In multiple chemical sensitivity syndrome, the source of the toxic exposure is not defined. One of the prominent features of this syndrome is chemical sensitivities, which means that even trace amounts of neurotoxins can provoke symptoms. With proper treatment, slow healing can take place and the degree of sensitivity can slowly recede. Early detection greatly increases the possibility of recovery. In severe cases, this condition can be debilitating.

The range of symptoms in chemical injury syndromes has

brought criticism and confusion in the medical community. The criticism appears to be tied to legal issues and potential lawsuits. The confusion appears to result from a poor understanding of how damage to the nervous system can affect the body systems it regulates and an inaccurate expectation that neurotoxic chemicals should behave like germs. Because chemical injuries are not diseases caused by a bacteria or virus, they do not follow a standard disease protocol.

Sometimes people confuse chemical sensitivities with allergies. There's a significant difference. When someone has an allergy, his immune system has an altered response to a harmless substance. (In technical terms, a traditional allergy is an IgE-mediated response and leads to hay fever symptoms.)

When a person or a few people have a chemical sensitivity, they are responding to a toxic poison sooner than other people. This should raise a red flag for the rest of the community. It could mean that while these few people are experiencing multiple chemical sensitivities and symptoms of neurotoxicity, others are developing cancers, neurodegenerative disorders, and disorders of the endocrine, immune, cardiovascular, or gastrointestinal systems.

Another increasingly reported and controversial syndrome is chronic fatigue syndrome. This syndrome is poorly understood, so we can't be sure of the role neurotoxic exposures play. In some cases, neurotoxic fatigue may be misdiagnosed as chronic fatigue syndrome. By reducing neurotoxic exposures (as discussed in the second half of this book) those with neurotoxic fatigue should experience significant improvement.

One of the theories is that a virus causes chronic fatigue syndrome. Neurotoxins could exacerbate a viral condition by interfering with immune functioning. A reduction in neurotoxic exposures allows the body to utilize its immune resources to fight off a viral attack rather than detoxify a neurotoxin.

Another prominent theory is that chronic fatigue syndrome is caused by decreased blood flow to the brain, a condition which is also seen in cases of neurotoxicity. People suffering from fatigue or chronic fatigue syndrome are likely to feel better after reducing neurotoxic exposures.

SUMMING IT UP

Neurotoxic chemicals play either a starring or supporting role in a long list of symptoms, diseases, and syndromes. In many of the conditions that may have multiple causes, the role of neurotoxicity is usually overlooked. For people who have been diagnosed with these conditions, reducing neurotoxic exposure is crucial.

If neurotoxins have been a causal factor, recovery will not be possible until the toxin is removed. If neurotoxins have played a supporting role, then reducing the neurotoxic burden on the body will increase the body's available resources. Neurotoxic exposures are a stressor to the body, depleting energy and diverting healing resources.

In some cases, neurotoxic chemicals cause direct damage to a specific organ. Besides damaging the brain, chemicals can also accumulate in the body's filtering systems—the kidney, liver, and lungs. These organs are particularly vulnerable to cancers because of the extended time they are in contact with toxins.

In other situations, neurotoxic chemicals contribute to a disease process. At the very least, they place a continual demand on bodily resources, which can lead to a state of exhaustion. According to the National Institute of Health, "the range of diseases which can be partially or completely initiated or caused by environmental factors is broad. The range includes, among other diseases: cardiovascular diseases; cancers; birth defects, malformations, and reproductive disorders; respiratory illness; deficiencies in the immune system . . . ; allergies and hypersensitivity disorders; nervous system abnormalities; and diseases of other organs, especially all the excretory organs including the kidney, liver, and intestine. . . . The health impact is enormous."[26]

To predict which diseases or symptoms neurotoxic chemicals may cause would be like predicting the impact of an electrical surge on a computer. Sometimes we get lucky and the surge protector prevents damage. Sometimes the electrical surge burns out all the circuits and connections. Given the risk, most people work hard to protect their equipment.

In the final analysis, a valuable computer can be replaced; the invaluable human brain cannot.

CHAPTER FIVE

HOW CHEMICALS INTERACT IN YOUR BODY

At this point, you may be wondering why some people are significantly affected by neurotoxins while others don't seem to be affected at all. Why does one person eventually develop Alzheimer's disease, while someone else gets headaches? The reactions of chemicals within the body are complicated, but they are not random or mysterious. This chapter will teach you the principles that govern the impact of toxins in the body. Once you understand these principles, you will understand why these poisons can affect people so differently.

Diseases caused by germs follow a specific course, and we can predict how germs will affect the body. We know that the hemolytic streptococci bacteria will cause a painful strep throat, and that the pox virus will cause chicken pox.

Chemicals are not germs. They do not cause a "sickness" in the sense that bacteria and viruses cause sicknesses. Whenever neurotoxins accumulate in the body more rapidly than they are excreted, they cause cell injury, which can lead to disease.

When you think about neurotoxicity in terms of an injury, you can understand how it affects people differently. For example, if you were to learn that two cars collided, you wouldn't be surprised to hear that one person walked away with bruises while another suffered a broken back. You wouldn't label it "bruise syndrome" and "broken back syndrome." You'd say the people had specific injuries resulting from the car accident.

There are predictable factors that influence injuries in a car accident: the speed of each car, which parts of the cars collided, the build of each car, whether passengers were sitting in the front seat or the back, whether they were wearing seat belts, and so on. If you knew these details, you could probably predict how serious the injuries would be.

In the same way, when people are injured by neurotoxic chemicals, there are predictable factors that influence the location and severity of their injury. These factors follow a logical pattern. In fact, you probably know more about these factors than you realize. For example, if you know anything about how alcohol affects people, you already understand some of the important factors that influence chemical injury. Based on what you know, answer the following question: How many beers would it take for someone to get drunk?

❖ Would it make a difference if the person were large or small? Male or female? A nine-year-old child?

❖ What if the person drank a shot of vodka a half-hour before drinking the beer?

❖ Would the effect be the same if the person took sleeping pills?

❖ Would your estimation be different if you knew the person drank a six-pack every night? If the person were a recovering alcoholic? Never drank at all?

To answer these questions accurately, you would have to consider the following factors: individual differences, bioaccumulation, synergy, and adaptation. These are the principles that help us predict how toxic chemicals will cause injuries. Let's take each factor one at a time.

INDIVIDUAL DIFFERENCES

Some of the factors that make one person more vulnerable than another include size, gender, age, state of health, nutritional status, genetics, and prior exposures to the substance. When two people are exposed to the same quantity of a substance, pound for pound, the smaller person has a larger exposure. You would expect a jockey to get drunk on less alcohol than a professional football player. Size difference is one of the reasons children are more vulnerable to chemical exposures than adults.

In our beer example, you probably predicted that a nine-year-old child would become intoxicated sooner than an adult. In addition to the difference in size, children are also more vulnerable to neurotoxins because their bodies are still growing and developing.

Gender plays a role in vulnerability to toxins. Women are more vulnerable than men. The fact that women tend to be physically smaller accounts for part of the difference, as does the fact that women tend to have a higher percentage of body fat. Hormonal factors also play a role. Certain neurotoxins pose an increased risk to women because they mimic the activity of estrogen (see chapter 2). When these toxic chemicals, known as xenoestrogens, trigger estrogen responses, they can set up a chain reaction with serious consequences. The full extent of the damage from these false messengers is not yet known.

State of health prior to an exposure is a factor in the risk of neurotoxic injury. If you're healthy and well nourished, you're better equipped to detoxify chemicals. Poor eating habits, lack of exercise, illness, and emotional stress all make a person more vulnerable to the effects of neurotoxicity.

The elderly tend to be vulnerable to toxins, particularly if they are in poor health. People who have been exposed to toxic chemicals for a lifetime can accumulate toxins in their bodies and may not have the capacity to detoxify from future exposures. The accumulation of toxins (called bioaccumulation) can increase the risk of dementia or cancer.

BIOACCUMULATION

In the next chapter, you will learn how the body gets rid of or detoxifies neurotoxic chemicals. If toxins enter faster than the body is able to excrete them, the body stores the toxins in fat or bone. This storage, or accumulation, of chemicals is called bioaccumulation. As long as the toxin remains in the body, it can resurface and cause future problems. This phenomenon is not unlike our municipal toxic dump sites, which eventually leak their toxins back into the air and water.

Most of us have personal experience with a similar principle— the "bioaccumulation" of calories. You may have noticed that one chocolate chip cookie will not make you gain weight. On the other hand, two boxes of them will. You've probably also observed that fat from potato chips and fat from chocolate chip cookies both have a similar effect—hip or waistline expansion.

Someone who has an accumulation of neurotoxins is more vulnerable to the next exposure. When factory owners and government agencies set standards on the use of neurotoxins in industrial settings, they need to remember the important principle of bioaccumulation. A worker may be able to work with a solvent for a certain period of time without any problems, but over time the toxin can accumulate to a level that causes serious cell injury. Switching from one neurotoxic substance to another is not a solution, because the body has to use similar resources to detoxify from any neurotoxin. Changing neurotoxins would be similar to switching from beer to wine to whiskey: they all cause intoxication.

When scientists perform animal studies on the toxicity of different chemicals, they ignore the important principle of bioaccumulation. They test a single chemical on laboratory rats and then get fresh stock before testing the next chemical. Human workers, on the other hand, may be required to use one neurotoxic chemical after another.

Some chemicals, such as alcohol, detoxify from the body in a relatively short period of time. Other chemicals remain in the body much longer. Chlordane, a chemical used to prevent termites under houses, has been detected in people ten years after a significant exposure.[1] Lead can actually be incorporated into the bone in place of calcium. Sometimes it remains for a lifetime, sometimes it reenters circulation. The body will pull lead back into circulation when it needs calcium. As it tries to pull calcium reserves from the bone, it gets lead instead. This is particularly hazardous to women and infants—times when the body needs calcium most are during pregnancy, breast-feeding, and menopause.[2]

SYNERGY

Synergy refers to the fact that combinations of chemicals can create new and more potent effects. That is, when the presence of one chemical increases the toxicity of a second chemical, there is synergy. In our beer example, you were asked if combining beer with sleeping pills would have an effect. In terms of math, synergy in this example would change a 4 + 4 equation into a 4 x 4 equation.

When people combine strong cleaning solutions containing bleach and ammonia they can create a synergistic effect. Malathion, an organophosphate pesticide, is synergistic with other chemicals. Malathion has been used in many cities for mosquito control and was sprayed aerially over most of California to control the Mediterranean fruit fly. Malathion is considered to be less toxic than other organophosphate pesticides, but its presence increases the toxicity of other chemicals, particularly other pesticides.[3] When citizens voice concern over the use of malathion in their communities, they are told it has low toxicity. They are not told about its dangerous synergistic effects.

Scientific studies of single chemicals on animals do not account for synergy. Anyone who understands synergy will question the legitimacy of these studies because none of us lives in a chemical-free vacuum. We are regularly exposed to multiple chemicals—cleaning products, cosmetics, chemicals in tap water, air pollution, car exhaust. That's why it's important to learn how to reduce neurotoxic chemicals in our homes to reduce their synergistic effects.

ADAPTATION

Sometimes people find that the longer they're exposed to a noxious substance the less it seems to bother them. In our beer example, you may have estimated that the person who drinks a six-pack every night has a higher tolerance (adaptation) for alcohol than someone who never drinks. Adaptation is the body's method of coping with repeated exposure to a toxin.

Our bodies are able to make a healthy adjustment to many conditions. We can adjust to climate changes, time changes, and increased physical activity, but our bodies never adjust to toxic substances. When a person is continually exposed to a neurotoxin, the symptoms of toxicity may subside. However, a lack of warning symptoms does not mean the body has stopped being dangerously affected, any more than turning off a fire alarm puts out a fire.

When the body is first exposed to a neurotoxin it will often respond with warning symptoms. With continued exposure the body will adapt to the poison to the best of its ability and the warning symptoms will disappear. This adaption, or tolerance, allows a person to continue functioning in spite of the poison, but this doesn't mean the substance is safe.

Perhaps the best example of this phenomenon is cigarette smoke. When someone first tries a cigarette, he may cough and choke, feel dizzy, and his lungs may ache. His body is trying to warn him that he's inhaling a toxin. If he persists in smoking, these warning signs will slowly disappear. His body will adapt to the continual onslaught of poison. This adaption will not, however, protect him from lung cancer, throat cancer, or other serious health problems.

Many people experience symptoms of withdrawal if the poison to which they've adapted is removed. Their bodies became so adept at surviving the poison that they have to readapt to living without it. For smokers, nerve cells throughout the entire body adjust to nicotine and then readjust when nicotine is removed. When someone stops smoking, his body begins to detoxify from the poison, and he may feel ill for as long as two weeks as the toxins leave his system.

Adaptation is a dangerous gift; it can lull us into thinking we're unaffected by the toxin. When the body is no longer able to adapt, we encounter painful or even fatal consequences.

෴

How people respond to toxic exposure varies from person to person. That's because individual differences, bioaccumulation, synergy, and adaptation determine the extent of a chemical injury. When two workers are standing next to each other on an assembly line and are exposed to the same chemical, they may not have the same physiological response. One worker might be larger than the other, one might have a cold, one might be a smoker, one might have been exposed to pesticides at home, one might be standing closer to the chemical, or there may be some other factor that alters the effect of the exposure.

The potential combinations of these factors can be complex, but they are not random or mysterious. This complexity should not be used to excuse the lack of medical knowledge about neurotoxins. Chemical injuries can and need to be clearly understood and rationally treated.

CHAPTER SIX

THE ROUTE CHEMICALS TAKE THROUGH YOUR BODY

How do dangerous neurotoxins get into our bodies? There are three routes of entry: the skin, the lungs, and the intestinal tract. When your skin is exposed to toxins, you may show symptoms such as a rash, dry skin, and burning eyes. When you inhale toxins you may cough, wheeze, and have difficulty breathing. When you ingest a toxin, you may experience nausea, cramping, and diarrhea.

ENTRY ROUTES

The Skin

Skin is your most effective barrier against foreign substances. If you put a drop of water on your skin, the water stays on the surface. If you rub it in, the droplet disperses, but the water still remains on the outside of the skin. Your skin can keep water-soluble substances outside of your body for a considerable period of time.

If you put a drop of lotion on your skin and rub it in, the lotion will quickly absorb. Lotion is able to penetrate the skin because it is lipid-soluble, which means it dissolves in fat rather than water. *Lipid* is a biological term for *fat*.

Lipids are an important part of your cells. The membrane, or outside, of a cell is made of a two-layer lipid coating. Lipids also give substance and structure to the inner part of the cell. A lipid-soluble substance can dissolve through the outside coating and penetrate the inside of the cell, both of your skin cells and the cells inside your body.

Many toxins, particularly those that affect the nervous system, are lipid-soluble. When a lipid-soluble chemical comes in contact with your skin, it is absorbed directly into your bloodstream. When you're at rest, blood travels through your entire body once each minute. When you're active, blood can circulate as many as six times each minute.[1] This means that toxins which enter through your skin can be rapidly circulated by the bloodstream to any part of your body.

You'd think that touching a chemical would be less dangerous than ingesting it. This isn't always the case. A chemical that enters through your digestive tract is filtered by the liver before it reaches general circulation,[2] while a chemical that enters through your skin enters directly into general circulation and can affect your body immediately.

It's critical to thoroughly wash your skin if hazardous chemicals come in contact with it, because more of the toxin is absorbed into the bloodstream and distributed throughout the body with each passing second. Chemistry labs and industrial plants that handle hazardous chemicals are equipped with showers to prevent lethal skin absorption in an accidental spill.

The direct entry through skin to the bloodstream can be beneficial with some types of medicines. Medications in the form of patches are used to distribute nitroglycerin and the hormone estrogen. Nicotine can be administered in a patch to help someone stop smoking, and medicine for motion sickness also comes in patch form. This allows the medicine to impact the body before being filtered by the liver or kidney.

The Digestive Tract
Chemicals that are swallowed could be distributed throughout your body using the same mechanisms that distribute food and water. But when you ingest chemicals, your cells begin the process of metabolism—biotransformation—to try to transform the toxin into a form your body can safely excrete. Chemicals that enter your body through

ingestion are filtered by the liver before they leave the blood vessels of the digestive system and enter your body's main bloodstream. The initial biotransformation is a crucial process because a toxin with direct access to the liver or kidney can cause permanent organ damage and leave your body unable to filter waste products or toxins in the future.

The Lungs

Chemicals that are inhaled enter your lungs and are transferred to the bloodstream through the oxygen exchange mechanism. Under normal conditions, 9 percent of your blood supply is in your lungs, exchanging carbon dioxide for oxygen.[3] Chemicals that pass through your lungs have direct access to your bloodstream. Like chemicals that enter through the skin, inhaled chemicals are not filtered by the kidney or liver until they are pumped through the body to reach these filter stations.

An additional danger from inhaled chemicals is that after the blood is oxygenated in the lungs, a portion of it is pumped directly to the brain.

There are two filters between the outside air and your brain. The first filter is your lungs. Any chemical that passes through your lungs has entered your body. The second filter is called the blood-brain barrier. This prevents many poisons from entering your brain, particularly water-soluble compounds.[4] Because neurotoxic compounds are lipid-soluble, they can cross this barrier.

Lipid-soluble toxins that enter the body through inhalation have direct brain access. Inhalant abuse, such as sniffing glues or octane boosters, causes an immediate high. Inhalant abuse poses a high risk of brain damage because of the quantity of neurotoxins that reach the brain. Smoking any substance produces fast results because of the easy access to the brain provided by the lungs.

WHAT HAPPENS INSIDE THE BODY

When a toxin enters your body, which route of entry poses the greatest threat? It depends on the toxic substance. All three routes can result in serious injury or death. For example, the "high" from illegal drugs may be different when the drug is sniffed, smoked, injected, or swallowed, but each of these routes affect the body and the brain.

Biotransformation

Once a toxic chemical has entered your body through any route of entry, your body works to protect you from injury. This process is called detoxification. Successful detoxification occurs when the chemical is excreted. For this to occur, the toxin has to be transformed into a substance your body can safely excrete.

Your body chemically changes—metabolizes—toxins the same way it metabolizes food. When a toxin is being metabolized, however, the process is called biotransformation. The transformed or metabolized product is known as a metabolite. Successful biotransformation turns a lipid-soluble neurotoxin into a water-soluble metabolite your body can excrete. Unsuccessful biotransformation creates a metabolite that is more dangerous than the original toxin.

Biotransformation occurs at a cellular level. The endoplasmic reticulum (a structure within the cell) contains enzymes that break down substances and rearrange their molecular form. There are two phases of biotransformation. Phase I reactions include oxidation (combining with an oxygen molecule), hydrolysis (the molecular bond is split and a hydrogen cation and the hydroxide anion of water are added), and reduction (removing an electron). These reactions are achieved by adding or removing an electron. Some toxins can be excreted following this process, while others are prepared for a Phase II reaction.

Phase II reactions consist of conjugation or synthesis. They can occur in the endoplasmic reticulum or in the cytoplasm (main body) of the cell. In this process, the toxin is bound to a protein. Once the toxin is bound, it is more easily excreted and has less ability to cause injury to the cells. The body is not safe from the toxin, however, until the toxin is excreted, because a bound toxin can be unbound and continue to wreak havoc.

Here's how the body detoxifies—biotransforms the ethonal—after ingesting beer.

Step 1: The ethanol (the alcohol part) is oxidized in a Phase I reaction in the endoplasmic reticulum. It becomes acetaldehyde.

Step 2: The acetaldehyde is oxidized in another Phase I reaction and becomes acetic acid.

Step 3: Acetic acid is conjugated (bound to a protein) in a Phase II reaction.

Step 4: The bound acetic acid can now be excreted from the body.[5]

Biotransformation is not always successful at reducing the toxicity of a substance. For example, the industrial chemical bromobenzene undergoes biotransformation in the liver to become bromobenzene epoxide, a substance that is highly toxic to the liver. If the amount of bromobenzene epoxide is small enough, the liver can further biotransform it into other metabolites that can be excreted safely. If the amount of bromobenzene epoxide is more than the liver's capacity, the epoxide will damage and kill the cells of the liver. An injury to the liver reduces the body's ability to detoxify future toxins or bodily waste products.[6]

Your body is more likely to make toxic metabolites when it's depleted of resources like enzymes, vitamins, minerals, and trace elements. These resources are depleted by previous toxic chemicals, poor nutrition, illnesses, and stress. Good nutrition can help replenish these resources and increase your body's ability to complete the biotransformation process successfully.

If a cell is unsuccessful in the biotransformation process, the toxin can permanently injure the cell. One of the cell's internal structures is the mitochondria, the cell's source of energy (ATP). If the mitochondria is damaged, the cell's future functioning will be impaired. Another critical structure in the cell is the nucleus, or control center. The nucleus contains the cell's DNA structure—its genetic code. Every cell in your body has the same DNA code.

A change to the DNA code can have devastating consequences. If the cell is unable to repair the damage to the DNA, it may reproduce mutated versions of itself. These mutations are thought to be the earliest stages of cancer.

Neurotoxins differ in their mutagenicity (ability to produce mutations). Some mutations have implications for the next generation because they can cause birth defects or miscarriages. It isn't known what percent of chromosomal abnormalities in newborns are the result of neurotoxins. In addition to cancer and birth defects, altered DNA may play a role in causing autoimmune diseases (see chapter 4).

While your liver is the primary source of biotransformation, any cell in your body is able to biotransform a toxin because biotransformation uses a cell's metabolism mechanisms. All cells metabolize nutrients from the blood supply, which delivers the substances needed for life and removes waste products. When the energy allocated for metabolism is spent on toxic chemicals instead of nutrients, the cell's resources are diverted from supplying its own needs.

If a toxin enters through the intestinal tract, the cells in the digestive system will biotransform the toxin before sending it to the liver for further detoxification. Biotransformation prevents the toxic substance from moving about freely in the blood plasma and causing cell damage throughout the body. This initial biotransformation is also important because it protects the liver from a toxic overload. This diverts the cells, however, from their primary function of digesting food.

Energy Depletion
Biotransformation requires a tremendous amount of energy! Your cells normally work to metabolize nutrients in the bloodstream into nutrients they can use. When your cells process a toxic chemical, they also expend energy, but they don't receive any nutrients.

Your nutritional state can impact your ability to detoxify. Some of the enzymes that break down toxins require the presence of certain vitamins or minerals to function effectively. If the vitamins and minerals aren't present, the body can't detoxify effectively. Even if they are present, nutritional reserves can be quickly depleted if you're overexposed to chemicals.

EXIT ROUTES

Chemicals can leave the body through perspiration, excretions from the bladder or bowels, or through exhalation. To a lesser degree, chemicals leave the body through breast milk, growing hair or nails, saliva, or even tears.

The kidneys play a major role in detoxification because excretion into the urine is thought to be the main exit route for toxins.[7] Toxins can also be excreted through bile when filtered by the liver.

Toxins released through sweat or breath can cause a foul odor. At some time you've probably smelled alcohol on someone's breath. This obvious exit route for detoxification is why police use breathalyzers to test the alcohol level in drivers under the influence. Often the breath and sweat of smokers has a foul odor as their bodies detoxify. People who work around chemicals may have a similar experience.

BIOACCUMULATION

Sometimes a neurotoxic exposure is greater than a person's capacity to detoxify. When biotransformation and detoxification processes get bogged down, neurotoxins accumulate in the body. This storage is your body's way of preventing dangerous toxins from circulating throughout your bloodstream and causing cell injury.

The most common storage site for lipid-soluble toxins is in lipid, or fat reserves. The primary fat reserves in the body are in the adipose tissue (adipose is another name for fat) and in the liver. Stored neurotoxins will remain in fat cells as long as there is a high level of neurotoxins in the blood. When the blood toxicity levels decrease, the stored neurotoxins can be released into the bloodstream for biotransformation and excretion. The storage, or accumulation, of toxins in the body is called bioaccumulation.

Storage is only a temporary solution for an overworked system unable to meet detoxification demands. The fat cell can release the toxin when calories are needed—during fasting or dieting, exercise, or high-demand situations. Heat exposure is also thought to release neurotoxins. When toxins are stored in the fat, they can surface whenever and wherever the fat reserves are being used.

Fat deposits perform important functions in the body. They store nutrients and they're used as building blocks for the structure of your cells. Without lipids, the insides of your cells would be liquid. Lipids also serve an important function in the brain: They provide insulation for the electrical activity of the nerve cells. You've probably heard of "gray matter" and "white matter" in the brain. Gray matter is the neurons; white matter is the lipid insulation around their axons.

So now you see the problem. When your body is overwhelmed by neurotoxic chemicals, it stores the toxins in fat cells until it can process them. In the meantime, these fat cells may get used in the body. Worst of all, the fat cells storing the neurotoxin could get used in the most important and the most vulnerable part of your body—your brain.

FROM MOTHER TO INFANT

For pregnant women, there's another route by which neurotoxins leave the body: from mother to developing baby. Like the blood-brain barrier, the placental barrier is very effective against water-soluble neurotoxins, but it's not impermeable to lipid-soluble neurotoxins.

One of the ways researchers monitor neurotoxins is to measure blood levels of chemicals in large numbers of people. As a group, women who are pregnant and breast-feeding have the lowest blood levels of pesticides. Where did the pesticides go? Since lipid-soluble neurotoxins pass through the placenta or breast milk, the toxic bio-accumulation of a mother will move into her baby.[8]

Not all neurotoxins are stored in fat. For example, the body handles neurotoxic lead by storing it in the bone in place of calcium. During pregnancy and breast-feeding, the mother's body provides the nutrients her baby needs. To provide calcium, the mother's body will pull it from her own bones. When lead has been stored in the bone in place of calcium, the baby will receive neurotoxic lead instead of the nutrient. Fetuses exposed to moderate to high levels of lead are more likely to be born with minor abnormalities and to have lower intelligence and increased behavioral problems.

～

Neurotoxins pose a risk to your body from the time they enter until they have been successfully excreted. They can cause irritation at the point of entry, resulting in rashes, coughing, or nausea. They can damage cells during biotransformation, which can lead to cancer or birth defects. They can accumulate and cause injury to a filter organ, such as the liver, lungs, and kidneys. If they're stored in your body, they can cause neurotoxic symptoms or disease. Neurotoxins can deplete your body of resources, making you more vulnerable to future toxic exposures or germs.

CHAPTER SEVEN

NEUROTOXICITY IN CHILDREN

Neurotoxins can harm the most vulnerable person of all: a developing baby. At low levels of exposure, neurotoxins can cause lower birth weight, learning problems, hyperactivity, and behavioral problems. Severe neurotoxicity during pregnancy can cause death, mental retardation, or birth defects. This is a distressing topic, but we need to learn about it. Our children's welfare depends on it.

BIRTH DEFECTS AND MENTAL RETARDATION

We've learned through human tragedy that chemicals which have no effect on an adult can have devastating consequences on a developing baby. The drug thalidomide was safely used by adults in Europe and Canada, but the children of mothers using thalidomide were born with deformed or missing arms or legs.

A Japanese factory that released methylmercury into the ocean in the 1950s created a human laboratory of neurotoxicity in the tiny fishing community of Minamata, Japan. The first sign of poisoning showed up in cats near the fishing docks. People spoke about the "dancing cats," until humans who ate large quantities of the contaminated fish began the same rigid, jerking muscle movements. This town, filled with neurotoxic tragedies, showed the world how highly toxic pollution affects humans.

The consequences of this tragedy continued into the next generation. Women who didn't have any symptoms of mercury poisoning gave birth to severely retarded children. In adults, methylmercury damage was primarily limited to the motor and visual cortex in the brain, so that muscular coordination and vision were affected.[1] In the developing child, the damage occurred throughout the entire brain. This incident made clear that a woman does not have to experience neurotoxic symptoms for neurotoxins to harm her child, and it shows that neurotoxins cause more damage to a developing infant than to an adult.

The reason neurotoxins are so dangerous during pregnancy is that they can prevent the normal development of the baby's nervous system. In the womb, each of the baby's organs develops in a specific sequence. If a toxin interferes when a particular organ is developing, that organ may not have a second chance to make up for lost growth. The nervous system is no exception. In the developing brain, the nervous system is developing its network of communication. Axons have to connect nerve cells to other nerve cells and to muscles or organs. If the axons cannot make their connections, the damage is permanent.

The communication of the nervous system depends on specific nerve pathways. We could compare the developing nervous system to laying railroad tracks. Just as a train can go only where tracks have been laid, the nerve cells can send communication only where axons can be successfully established. One condition believed to interfere with axon development is Fetal Alcohol Syndrome (FAS). Children born with FAS tend to have mild mental retardation and growth deficiencies.[2] This is why many liquor and grocery stores have signs warning women not to drink alcohol during pregnancy.

Severe toxic exposures, such as at Minamata, are not the only cause of neurotoxic injuries in children. Minor birth defects and neurological injuries can occur at lower levels of neurotoxic exposure. Some of these neurotoxins have a lifetime effect, even after they can no longer be detected in the body.[3] For this reason, more research on the effects of air and water pollution on infants and children is critical.

One set of researchers has done extensive work on the effects of the heavy metal lead on children. Usually when people think of a lead exposure, they think of lead-based paints or the lead in pipes leaching into water. Leaded gasoline emits lead into the air.

Over a two-year period, these researchers measured the level of lead exposure in over 11,000 babies born in a Boston hospital by measuring the lead in the blood of the umbilical cord. This study traced an environmental pollutant to the lifeline of the developing baby. What they found was a significant correlation between the level of lead in the umbilical cord and the monthly sales figures of the gasoline additive alkyl lead in the state of Massachusetts.

Based on the amount of lead in the blood, the babies were classified as having low, medium, or high lead exposure. Babies with a medium exposure were twice as likely to have minor abnormalities as the babies with low lead exposure. Babies with high lead exposure were three times more likely to have minor abnormalities.[4] This study demonstrated that babies exposed to higher levels of a neurotoxin were more likely to be born with minor abnormalities.

LEARNING AND BEHAVIORAL PROBLEMS

We don't currently know how many cases of learning disabilities, hyperactivity, attention deficit disorder (ADD), behavioral problems, and emotional problems in children are the result of neurotoxicity. We also don't know how many cases are made worse by neurotoxins. We do know that neurotoxins can alter behavior and learning.

Children can't express their experiences the way adults can. A young child won't say, "I need a nap." Instead, she'll act out her need for rest by crying, screaming, fighting with siblings, or demanding things. Every parent knows that to monitor a young child's health and well-being, you monitor behavior. When a baby is sick, he screams; he doesn't say, "Pardon me, Mom, I have an earache."

As time passes, a child learns how to walk, talk, coordinate hands and fingers, read, understand numbers, make friends, and learn a multitude of other tasks. This is when neurological deficits become apparent.

Mild to moderate neurotoxicity in a child is most likely to express itself in learning or behavioral problems. Minor neurotoxic injuries that affect learning usually don't become apparent until the child is older and attempts complex tasks.

Although most of the scientific research about the lifelong effects of neurotoxic chemicals during pregnancy have been performed on animals, these studies give us important clues about how neurotoxins can affect children. In animals, neurotoxins have been found to cause lowered birth weights, hyperactivity, behavioral problems, and problems with learning.[5]

Consider this example of just one animal study. Mice who were exposed to low levels of PCB's around the time of birth responded slowly to new or stressful situations, and they had problems adjusting to a new environment.[6]

Now, the social demands on a mouse are considerably less than the demands on a child. Think about what would happen to a child who responded slowly to a new or stressful environment. How would this child do in a classroom? A child who learns just a bit slower or who slows down in the presence of stress or novelty would be at a tremendous disadvantage. When children fall behind in basic skills, the gap between their performance and the performance of others can increasingly widen.

The Boston researchers who studied the effects of lead on newborns also studied the effects of lead on school children. Because our bodies store lead in bone, these researchers collected baby teeth from over three thousand first- and second-graders to find out how much lead they had been exposed to. When children with high levels of lead were compared to children with low levels, they were found to have lower IQs, lower verbal skills, lower auditory and language performance, and they scored lower on a measure of attention. The researchers also asked the teachers to rate the behavior of the children in the classroom. Those with high levels of lead were rated as more distractible, less organized, and their overall functioning was rated below their peers.[7]

It's no coincidence that as neurotoxins in air, water, and food increase, the number of children with learning disabilities, attention deficits, hyperactivity, behavioral problems, and emotional disturbances also increases. These are the types of neurological disturbances we can predict in children with low-level neurotoxic poisoning.

In addition to controlling learning and behavior, the brain is the center of emotion and self-control. There are specific brain structures that control emotion, the ability to organize information, and the ability to plan ahead. These skills are the foundation upon which a child builds self-control. A neurotoxic injury to these regions could cause an emotional disturbance.

A growing number of children with behavioral and learning problems have significantly improved or completely recovered when neurotoxic chemicals were removed from their homes and diets. Many of these children also suffer from asthma, allergies to foods, allergies to pollens and molds, ear infections, and other chronic infections. It's not clear how the combination of allergies and neurotoxins are related, but it's possible for a neurotoxic injury to alter immune functioning (see chapter 4) and predispose a child to allergies or repeated infections. It's also possible that a child with allergies, asthma, or repeated infections may be more vulnerable to the effects of neurotoxic chemicals.

Some pediatricians and allergists have been highly successful in treating these types of cases by reducing neurotoxic exposures, eliminating certain food additives and foods from the child's diet, treating the child for other allergies, identifying nutritional deficits, and strengthening the immune system. These treatments have allowed many children to lead healthy lives. In some cases, children diagnosed with hyperactivity, ADD, and behavioral problems have been helped or cured without the use of Ritalin or other drugs.[8]

Since there haven't been many scientific studies on the effectiveness of these treatments, some doctors are skeptical about their outcome. But parents with children who are severely affected don't have time to wait for scientists to get interested in doing research. Many parents have been able to help their children by aggressively seeking these alternative treatments.

The potential role of a neurotoxic injury or some type of allergy should be considered when a child shows unaccountable changes in learning, behavior, or activity levels. If these changes only occur at certain times of the day, or certain times of the year, it would be worthwhile to investigate whether the child is being exposed to neurotoxic chemicals or whether some type of food or inhalant allergy is present.

Children who have been injured by neurotoxins before or after birth may have to learn to compensate for minor neurological deficits. As increasing numbers of children are being diagnosed with learning disabilities, many school systems are providing services to help children compensate for difficulties in learning. For children with behavioral problems, parents will want to get specific training in effective behavioral techniques to give their child the best chance of gaining self-control. Children who've been injured by neurotoxins will benefit from parents who help them gain skills and give them confidence that they can succeed. Parents can help children conquer any type of deficit, injury, or illness.

It's important for all children to be protected from neurotoxins in our homes and in our schools to allow them to grow, learn, and develop. This protection becomes especially important for children who have already been injured by a neurotoxic exposure, because they will be more vulnerable to future neurotoxic injuries.

∽

As the use of neurotoxins in our air, water, and food increases, large numbers of children are being diagnosed with learning disabilities, hyperactivity, attention deficits, and behavioral problems—the very types of neurological disturbances we can predict in children with low levels of neurotoxic poisoning. While education experts get more adept at diagnosing learning disabilities, and doctors fill prescriptions for Ritalin, industries continue to produce billions of dollars of neurotoxins. Within industry, experts look at cost/benefit ratios. Is any benefit worth these costs to our children?

CHAPTER EIGHT

WHY IS NEUROTOXICITY USUALLY UNDETECTED?

Why is the connection between neurotoxic chemicals and serious health hazards virtually unknown? Because as consumers, we have not been provided with accurate information about health risks from products that contain neurotoxins.

Common household products and cosmetics do not list warning symptoms of neurotoxicity; these substances are not even identified as neurotoxins. Most of us falsely assume that since these products are sold in grocery stores, they've met some type of safety standard. We have no regulation over the use of toxins in our homes and no health inspector comes to measure levels of toxic fumes.

The World Health Organization reported in 1986, "[It] is not known how often insidious problems of neurotoxicity may lie undetected because effects are incorrectly attributed to other conditions (advancing age, mood disorders) or misdiagnosed. The early and incipient stages of intoxication produced by environmental agents are frequently marked by vagueness and ambiguity . . . thus the potential is large for the occurrence of subtle, undetected effects, which nonetheless have an important bearing on the quality of life."[1]

Many chemical injuries do not show up immediately. The longer the time between a neurotoxic exposure and the symptoms of a neurotoxic injury, the more difficult it is to make the connection. A chemical injury to an infant that alters the child's ability to learn will not be apparent until the child is older. Some injuries that occur during pregnancy or infancy are not apparent until puberty or adulthood.

For example, the food additives MSG and NutraSweet have been linked in infant animals with damage to an area of the brain called the hypothalamus. A similar injury in a human infant would likely result in obesity and neuroendocrine disturbances, such as low levels of certain hormones and reproductive failure. The neuroendocrine disorders would not be apparent until puberty or adulthood (when trying to conceive a child).[2] How could a couple know if they were unable to conceive a child because one of them was injured by MSG as a toddler? How could someone who suffered from obesity know if the cause was MSG in baby food?

Unawareness leads to the greatest risk of neurotoxic exposure. Did you know that a freshly painted, newly carpeted room to welcome the new baby may look great, but it can also expose the child to a variety of solvents and petrochemicals? (Chapter 17 discusses less toxic options.) Potentially, the same thing happens to us every day. If you've ever been at a standstill in heavy traffic and started to get a headache, fall asleep, or suddenly felt very angry, you may have been experiencing a neurotoxic reaction to gasoline fumes. When an office is sprayed for bugs and half the employees go home with the "flu," the company and the employees are paying the price of neurotoxicity.

Many people want to know which single neurotoxin is the most dangerous. This is like asking which single alcoholic beverage will get a person drunk. The most dangerous chemical for you is the neurotoxin you are being exposed to. When you're not informed about how to associate symptoms of neurotoxicity with the use of a toxic product, you're at risk.

MEDICINE: MEDICAL PERSONNEL LACK TRAINING

We expect doctors to be informed and trained in issues of health. Unfortunately, medical personnel are not adequately trained in neurotoxicity. While a heart surgeon may be well qualified to perform a coronary artery bypass, he may not know the role of pesticides or other neurotoxins in high blood pressure, which increases the risk of heart disease. Someone with neurotoxic symptoms of headaches, vision problems, fatigue, and depression could get referred to several specialists—an eye doctor for the vision, a neurologist for the headaches, and a psychiatrist for the depression and fatigue. These specialists would not necessarily be trained in neurotoxicity.

In a survey of medical training facilities, the Texas Rural Health Field Services investigated the amount of training provided by medical schools, nursing programs, and veterinary programs in recognizing and treating cases of pesticide poisoning. This is an important question because of the number of people exposed to pesticides at work and in the home. According to the World Health Organization, "workers exposed to pesticides are one of the largest occupational populations at risk in the world."[3] About 1.1 billion pounds of pesticides are used each year in the U.S. In 1991, this averaged out to 4.3 pounds for every man, woman, and child.[4]

The medical training survey found that nursing schools provided almost no training on pesticide poisoning, and medical schools provided minimal training for doctors in how to diagnose or treat cases of pesticide poisoning. The legal and educational materials available were almost exclusively for professionals working with migrant farm workers. Veterinarians were found to be the group of medical professionals most qualified to diagnose and treat pesticide poisoning.[5]

The likelihood of a general practitioner in an urban setting having any training in recognizing or treating low-level, chronic pesticide exposures is slight. On the other hand, the likelihood that his patients are being exposed to pesticides is extremely high. Americans are estimated to apply some 300 million pounds of toxic pesticides in and around their homes each year. On average, suburban homeowners use more pesticides per acre than farmers use on their fields! Half of pesticide deaths occur in children, and 70 percent of poisonings involve children under the age of five.[6]

Almost the entire United States population is exposed to neurotoxic pesticides in their homes or on the job. In addition to agricultural workers, hospital personnel and workers in food industries are regularly exposed to pesticides. Office workers and homeowners encounter pesticides when they use bug spray or hire professional exterminators. Yet the medical community has abdicated its role in detecting or treating pesticide-related health problems. The fact is, traditional medicine has abdicated its role in the whole field of neurotoxicity. Research on neurotoxicity is primarily conducted by industry and regulatory agencies. Scientists in other health science disciplines, such as behavioral toxicology, neuropsychology, toxicology, and nutrition, are likely to be more qualified to speak to these issues than medical doctors.

THE GOVERNMENT: FAILURES IN REGULATION

Between 1979 and 1995, the Environmental Protection Agency (EPA) New Chemicals Program reviewed over 30,000 new chemical substances. Only four substances were judged an unreasonable risk and prohibited from being produced and distributed.

When a new substance is invented, a company must provide a ninety-day pre-manufacture notice (PMN). According to the EPA, less than half the PMN applications for new chemicals include any toxicological data. No testing at all may be required, depending on the quantity likely to be produced, the type of chemical, and projected releases. In the past decade, between 1,500 and 3,000 new chemicals were reviewed by the EPA each year.[7]

Once a chemical has been registered with the EPA, it's very hard to remove it from the approved list, no matter how much evidence exists about its toxicity to humans. The EPA had evidence in the 1970s that Alar (a chemical used to make apples ripen) posed a cancer risk, particularly to children, but they took no action until the public outcry of 1989. When the apple industry was threatened with plummeting sales because people were afraid of getting cancer from Alar, the EPA announced its intention to remove Alar. At the same time the EPA was working to ban the chemical because of its link to cancer in children, the public was assured that apples treated with Alar posed no threat. The government bought $15 million of the treated apples to distribute to schools, prisons, and aid programs.[8]

Even after a chemical is banned, it may still be produced. Chemicals banned in the U.S., such as DDT, can be produced legally in the U.S. and sold to other countries. While DDT has been banned in this country, food with DDT residues imported from other countries is routinely sold in our grocery stores.[9]

In 1992, toxic chemical waste generated by industry was reported to be 37.33 billion pounds. U.S. manufacturers reported releasing 3.18 billion pounds of toxic chemicals into the environment. Of this, 1.84 billion pounds were released into the air, 273 million pounds into surface water, 338 million pounds into land, 726 million pounds of toxic waste were injected underground, and 2.84 billion pounds were transferred offsite for recycling. Another 34 million pounds of toxic chemicals in waste were generated as a result of nonroutine accidents.[10]

Although people trust our regulatory agencies to test and regulate the use of toxic chemicals, these agencies are not fulfilling their role. In fact, sometimes these agencies can't even protect themselves. The Environmental Protection Agency (EPA) learned firsthand about neurotoxicity in October 1987. While re-carpeting 27,000 square yards of their building, 124 out of 2,000 employees were injured by neurotoxic chemicals in the carpeting and carpet glue.[11] One woman was taken to a hospital in respiratory collapse.

This was not the first such case. The EPA had received numerous requests to investigate this potent source of indoor air pollution. The EPA's tragic experience provided an almost perfect laboratory experiment to address this serious health hazard—employees whose work habits were already known were suddenly confronted with neurotoxic symptoms. Yet the EPA did not act to protect its workers. The injured EPA employees had to turn to their union for protection. It was the union that requested an investigation.

Union representatives testified before congressional committees in October 1988 and May 1989. In December 1989, the union filed a Toxic Substances Control Act section 21 petition. By March 1990, the union was unofficially told the reason their petition was denied: It could cost the carpet industry "billions of dollars."[12]

In April 1992, the Union was contacted by Anderson Labs in Dedham, Massachusetts. Dr. Rosalind Anderson is a physiologist with an independent laboratory who was investigating chemicals in carpet samples. To do this, she exposed mice to air blown over carpet samples and then measured the respiratory effects. Nothing happened, at first. But people who had been injured by carpeting learned about her research. They began to send her their carpet samples. Dr. Anderson was skeptical, but she was willing to use their samples.

The results were stunning! These carpet fumes worked like nerve gas on the mice. The mice gasped, turned blue, lost their balance, and suffered paralysis and lung hemorrhages. Within four hours many of them had died. In October 1992, Dr. Anderson did another study. This time, thirteen carpet samples were randomly purchased. Three of them had a fatal effect on mice.[13]

Still the EPA refused to take action to protect consumers or their own employees from neurotoxins in carpeting. An EPA official stated that "25% of carpet being a hazard is not enough to require a warning label on all carpets."[14]

The carpet industry announced a self-regulatory program in July 1992, called the "Green Tag Program." In September, the EPA Union filed a complaint with the Federal Trade Commission (FTC) and EPA, claiming that the Green Tag Program was fraudulent, endangering public health.[15] As of 1996, no action has been taken and it doesn't appear that any regulatory action is in the wings.

This tragic situation follows the typical scenario surrounding the current lack of protective regulations on toxic products:

1. A neurotoxic product for industrial and consumer use was allowed on the market.
2. As a result, people were seriously injured. (To date, some EPA employees are still unable to work at the renovated building, and others are able to work only by computer-links from their homes.)
3. Animal testing provided strong evidence that the product was neurotoxic, but the research was disregarded because it posed a threat to the industry.
4. The industry was given an opportunity to protect itself from legal retribution.
5. No regulatory action was taken.
6. The industry began a public relations campaign. (In this

case, they offered the "Green Tag Program," which experts
consider to be fraudulent.)
7. The public is not being protected.

Rather than address a serious health hazard, the EPA and the carpet industry did damage control on corporate image and public perception. The health of the industry was given higher priority than the
health of human beings.

This case also demonstrates the failure of governmental agencies to protect you and your family from neurotoxins. EPA employees are more knowledgeable about environmental regulations and
have better access to government action than employees in other
industries. If the EPA union can't motivate the EPA to take action,
what's it going to take?

When governmental agencies fail to regulate toxic chemicals,
people get injured. Unfortunately, children are often the first victims
of toxic injuries. Three years after the EPA building was recarpeted,
and two years before Dr. Anderson found that toxic carpeting caused
death in laboratory mice, a high school in Springfield, Virginia, was
recarpeted. Springfield is a suburb of Washington, D.C., not far from
the offices of the EPA. When the school was recarpeted in August
1990, they could not have anticipated the health problems that would
follow. During the fall and spring, there were numerous fainting inci-
dents. And while industry and governmental regulators continued to
debate over how much poison is poisonous, one of the students at
the recarpeted high school suddenly died.[16]

Cancer Tests Are Not Enough

As consumers, we must be well-informed about neurotoxins because
the government is not effective in regulating their use. Of the 70,000
chemicals registered with the EPA, few have actually undergone testing for neurotoxicity. Currently the EPA requires tests of neurotoxicity only on "high volume" substances, which means that over 80
percent of the registered chemicals will not be tested for neurotoxicity. Even pesticides that are specifically formulated to be neurotoxic
may not have to be tested for neurotoxicity.[17]

Are you shocked? You probably thought chemicals were

adequately tested before being sold, used in consumer products, and applied to our food. But most toxicity research has focused on cancer, not neurotoxicity.

Tests that measure cancer rates are inadequate to determine neurotoxicity. The fact that these so-called "tests" are touted to the public causes consumers to believe that products are being monitored for safety when they're not. Cancer is only the tip of the toxic iceberg. Let me illustrate just how inadequate cancer tests are for neurotoxins.

Suppose you were a scientist and you wanted to know whether vodka posed a threat to human health and behavior. What would you think about a study in which one hundred mice were exposed to vodka in their drinking water every day for ninety days and were then tested for cancers and tumors? How accurately do you think this study would reflect the effect of alcohol on humans? This study might demonstrate that vodka was not associated with cancer in laboratory mice, but once you knew that vodka was not a carcinogen (cancer causing agent), would you want someone to drink it while operating heavy machinery or running a table saw? Would you feel safe allowing vodka to be a part of a school lunch program?

This example may seem ludicrous, but when substances are registered without tests for neurotoxicity, they end up in the workplace and can end up in the classroom.

The chemical chlordane, which was sprayed under houses to prevent termites, has been characterized by the EPA as "a probable human carcinogen." Apart from any risk of cancer, chlordane is toxic to the liver, the nervous system, and the immune system. It has the potential to move into the bone marrow and damage T, B, and natural killer cells of the immune system as they are developing.[18] When researchers limit their work to the cancer-causing potential of a substance, their studies do not reveal neurotoxicity, because they don't look for it. Cancer studies can only report the statistical probability of cancer.

SCIENCE: UNDERESTIMATING THE REAL RISKS

Toxicologists are the scientists who study toxins. To put it technically, toxicology is the field of science that studies the adverse effects of chemicals on living organisms.[19] All of the substances toxicologists evaluate are poisonous, including the neurotoxins. Toxicologists agree that the toxic chemicals they study are fatal at some level, but they disagree over what quantity of each poison is dangerous.

This debate is very important to each of us, because the answers toxicologists come up with determine governmental regulatory standards. These standards determine which chemicals an employee can be exposed to on the job, which chemicals can be added to foods and medicines, which chemicals a city can spray for weed or pest control, and which products are sold in your grocery store. To understand whether or not the products we use are safe, we have to understand the language of toxicology.

Toxicology: The Science of Risk

Toxicologists work with probability. They are interested in the probability that a poisonous substance will actually cause harm. This probability is called risk, or hazard. Toxicologists do not focus on the intrinsic toxicity of the substance, they focus on risk—"the probability that injury will result from a chemical under specific conditions."[20] So this is the question toxicologists ask: "How likely is it that this poison will actually injure somebody?"

The job of toxicologists is to identify risk and to establish "safety." In the field of toxicology, the word *safety* does not actually mean safe. Toxicologists define safety as "the practical certainty that injury will not result from use of a substance under specified conditions of quantity and manner of use."[21] High safety means low risk, low safety means high risk. Whenever you hear about "safety," keep in mind that it's referring to the probability of an injury, not to something actually being safe.

When toxicologists calculate the risk or the probability of an event, they are working with yes/no types of questions. They ask questions like, Did the subject die or not? Did the subject get cancer or not? Were there birth defects or not?

These yes/no types of probabilities would be appropriate to use if you wanted to find out your chances of winning the lottery. They are not appropriate to calculate your health risk from neurotoxic chemicals because health is not a yes/no proposition. In between good health and death is a range of suffering which a yes/no probability cannot calculate: headaches, fatigue, infertility, memory loss, personality changes, and many other problems.

Within the field of toxicology, there are researchers who have recognized these limitations. These researchers began a new field of science in 1972 called behavioral toxicology. A behavioral toxicologist works with people, using neuropsychological tests to look at things like reaction time, memory, and problem-solving abilities.[22] Unlike mainstream toxicologists, they consider the symptoms reported by people who have been exposed to toxins to be an important source of information.

Another type of toxicology study is teratology. These studies investigate the effects of toxic chemicals on offspring. When a toxic chemical injures a child prenatally, it is called a teratological effect.

Determining Risk

To study the risk/safety of different substances, toxicologists use animal studies and epidemiology studies. The combination of information from both types of studies can compensate for the flaws of each. Epidemiology, from the word *epidemic,* studies the incidence, distribution, and control of diseases in the human population. These studies look at the effects of toxins in large groups of people. It was an epidemiology study which found that pregnant and breast-feeding women have the lowest blood levels of pesticides, indicating that the pesticides are passed to the infant through the placenta and through breast milk.

Epidemiology studies are used to determine which areas of the country have the highest rates of cancer. The information derived from epidemiology studies is important, but these studies are not conducted very often, and you can probably guess why: They're expensive. For this reason, most of the research is based in a laboratory.

Animal studies usually begin by establishing two limits for a toxin, the LD50 and the NOEL. The LD50 is an abbreviation for the lethal dose for 50 percent of the test animals and is one of the first standards established for each substance. At LD100, all the animals die. LD50s are measured by mg/kg, which means the milligrams of substance per kilogram of animal (or person). This LD50 measure is a standard measure, and it can be used as a basis of comparison between substances. For alcohol, the LD50 is 10,000 mg/kg, for

DDT it is 100 mg/kg, and for dioxin (TCDD) it is .001 mg/kg.[23] According to a toxicology textbook, "Lethality provides a measure of comparison among many substances whose mechanism and sites of action may be markedly different."[24]

In the LD50 phase of study, animals are observed for signs of toxicity, such as difficulty breathing, muscular weakness, tremors, and so on. These signs indicate which bodily systems are being affected.[25] These observations and the autopsies that follow help to establish specific target organs for the chemical studied. Toxicologists can learn if a substance is most likely to accumulate in the brain, liver, kidney, or some other organ.

The other important threshold value in toxicology is the NOEL. NOEL stands for "no observable effects level." The NOEL is the maximum amount of a toxin that can be administered to the animal without any observable symptoms.

Doses between the NOEL and the LD50 are used to establish a dose-response relationship. The theory is that as the amount of toxin increases, the severity of effects will also increase. Somewhere between the NOEL and the LD50 is an LOEL (lowest observable effect level) and an FEL (frank effect level).[26] At the LOEL, for example, an experimental animal might begin to have a slight tremor, whereas at the FEL he might begin to have convulsions. The dose-response relationship establishes a connection between an increased level of exposure and an increased risk of toxicity. It does not account for repeated low-level exposures to multiple toxins.

Interpreting the Language of Risk
You may be wondering whether this scale from NOEL to LD50 in animals accurately predicts the effects of neurotoxins in humans. That's a legitimate question. In fact, the experts agree there's a fundamental problem in animal studies. Toxicologists know that "on a body weight basis, man is generally more vulnerable than the experimental animal, probably by a factor of about 10."[27]

It's well known that different species of animals metabolize toxins differently. In fact, sometimes different strains of rats metabolize a toxin differently.[28] The reason rodents are routinely selected for toxicity studies is because they're cheap. They're not selected because they're the best animal representative of human metabolism.

Initial studies will not reveal the differences between animal metabolism and human metabolism. For example, rodents are able to quickly excrete the organophosphate pesticide leptophos (sold as Abar and Phosvel). In humans, leptophos accumulates in the tissues to a greater extent than most other organophosphate compounds.[29] Studies on rats with this pesticide do not reveal the high risk to humans. If monkeys are used in experiments with the food additive MSG, the human health hazard will be underestimated because monkeys do not accumulate MSG the way humans do. This makes them much less vulnerable than we are to its neurotoxic effects.[30]

Animal studies can accurately show that a substance is a toxin, and they can roughly estimate the amount of the toxin that is dangerous to people. Animal studies can also show which organs are most likely to be affected by a chemical, which chemicals are most likely to be passed from mother to offspring, and whether a chemical is neurotoxic. What animal studies cannot do is replace human studies.

Another important question in animal studies is the legitimacy of the NOEL (no observable effects level) measure. You know from personal experience that not all physical symptoms can be seen. For example, how could someone observe a headache in a rat? Yet NOEL implies that if it can't be observed, it didn't happen.

If a food additive caused a child's thinking to be impaired, what indication would be given by the rat? To take it further, what if this child's thinking is mildly impaired so that she has difficulty learning her multiplication tables, which leads to problems with her future mastery of math skills and later academic performance? Given that rats do not possess the skills and abilities that make us human, we have to question whether the NOEL for a rat is an acceptable measure of safety for humans.

At the other end of the dose-response relationship is the LD50 measure. This measure of risk of death does not account for quality of life or health. There's a broad range of human experiences between feeling good and being dead. The cost of repeated illnesses, chronic fatigue, lost abilities, and mental impairment cannot be easily calculated. Chemicals that contribute to many chronic conditions may not be fatal, but they rob us of vitality.

The nonfatal consequences of neurotoxicity in the lives of real people may not qualify as a statistic in a toxicology study. In fact, most of the consequences of toxic chemicals are never counted in risk/benefit equations for neurotoxins. But the lost intellectual potential of a child, the early dementia of a grandparent, or a couple's inability to conceive a child are the losses of real people. And for them, their families, and their friends, these losses are significant.

The most important factors *not* considered in the dose-response relationship are the consequences of multiple, chronic, and low-level toxic exposures for the population and the environment.

Multiple Exposures

In the real world we're exposed to multiple toxins on a daily basis. While our bodies detoxify from one chemical exposure, they may not have adequate resources to manage the second, third, or fourth toxin. Also, as discussed in chapter 5, some toxins act synergistically; the combined effect of two toxins may be much more toxic than the effect of each toxin added together. When a city uses malathion to control mosquitoes, for example, it doesn't calculate how malathion is synergistic and can make people more vulnerable to the other toxins in the environment.

Chronic Exposures

A chronic exposure is one that occurs continually or repeatedly. You are chronically exposed to the detergent you use to wash your clothes, the cosmetics products you put on your skin, and chemicals used every day at your job. A chronic exposure to a substance can have a different effect than an acute exposure (a single exposure to a substance or several exposures in a short time period).[31] Toxicology studies primarily measure acute toxicity, which is the immediate effect of a single exposure to the toxin. These studies do not account for a lifetime of repeated low-level exposures.

Low-Level Exposures

The dose-response relationship does not take into account low-level toxic poisoning—exposures to a small amount of a chemical usually considered to be irrelevant. When someone near you is wearing perfume, for example, you're exposed to a low level of the perfume. Intuitively, you would assume that a stronger concentration of a toxin is more poisonous than a weaker concentration. This assumption is the foundation of the dose-response relationship. It is not necessarily the case.

In a study of the pesticide aldicarb, it was found that 1 ppb (part per billion) in drinking water was more damaging to the immune system of mice than 1,000 ppb (parts per billion). The weaker dilution suppressed the immune response more than the stronger dilution.[32] That's not the result you would expect, but it's a well-known effect in toxicology. Toxicologists know that when a substance is ingested, a weaker solution of the substance tends to be more toxic than a concentrated solution.[33]

This makes sense when you think about it. If a person ate a teaspoon of poison, his body might be able to protect itself through vomiting or diarrhea. The threat would be so dangerous that the body would be alerted to respond. But if this person ingested only a few grains of poison, his body might not recognize the danger. With the lower concentration, more of the poison could actually reach his cells. The usual cell-repair mechanisms may not be triggered. As another example, some people find that they are physically unable to consume a large amount of very strong, undiluted liquor because of the defense mechanisms of the body: burning throat, throwing up, or passing out. If the strong liquor is diluted, however, they would be able to consume a large quantity of it.

The impact of low-level toxic exposures is the least understood and most poorly investigated of all neurotoxic phenomena. Preliminary research indicates that low-level exposures pose a significant, unrecognized health hazard.[34]

Risk in the Real World

Regulatory agencies make decisions about the use of chemicals based on probabilities generated by animal models of NOEL and LD50 levels. The Food and Drug Administration (FDA) is the regulatory agency over food additives and cosmetic products, and the Environmental Protection Agency (EPA) is the regulatory agency over most other chemicals, including pesticides. These agencies allow the use of toxic chemicals, but theoretically they regulate the amount so that the cancer risk ratios range from 1 in 10,000 to 1 in 100,000,000. The Occupational Safety and Health Administration (OSHA) is the regulatory agency for toxic chemicals used in the workplace. In general, OSHA will allow lifetime cancer risks of up to 1 in 1,000.[35]

The statistic of 1 in 1,000 or 1 in 100,000,000 appears to represent low risk. But is it realistic? Most of us don't know 100,000,000 people, but all of us know someone who has had cancer. In addition to the number of people you know with cancer, add the number of your relatives, friends, and acquaintances who've had Alzheimer's disease, Parkinson's disease, ALS, heart disease, high blood pressure, chronic fatigue, multiple chemical sensitivities, Gulf War syndrome, sick building syndrome, lupus, arthritis, miscarriages, premenstrual syndrome, hypothyroidism, learning disabilities, attention deficit disorder, repeated infections, and mysterious health problems that no doctor can explain or cure. Is it more than 1 in 1,000? Is it more than 1 in 100? Is it just too many?

Are We Human Guinea Pigs?

Despite the trappings of objective scientific inquiry and volumes of complex reports, the impact of toxic chemicals is poorly understood and poorly documented. The majority of chemicals are not tested at all. Most people do not realize just how much information on the health hazards of chemicals is nonexistent. When the National Research Council examined the need for information about health hazards of industrial and consumer chemicals in 1984, they found an overwhelming need for health hazard assessments and toxicity data for every class of chemical.

The council found there was no toxicity data or minimal data for 66 percent of pesticides, 81 percent of food additives, 84 percent of cosmetic ingredients, and 88-90 percent of chemicals in commerce.[36] This means they weren't able to perform even a partial health hazard assessment on 2,211 pesticide ingredients used on food, 6,988 food additives, 2,864 cosmetic ingredients, and over 42,700 chemicals used in commerce. (See figure 8.1 on next page.)

The majority of neurotoxicity testing in the workplace occurs after workers are seriously injured, not as a preventive measure.

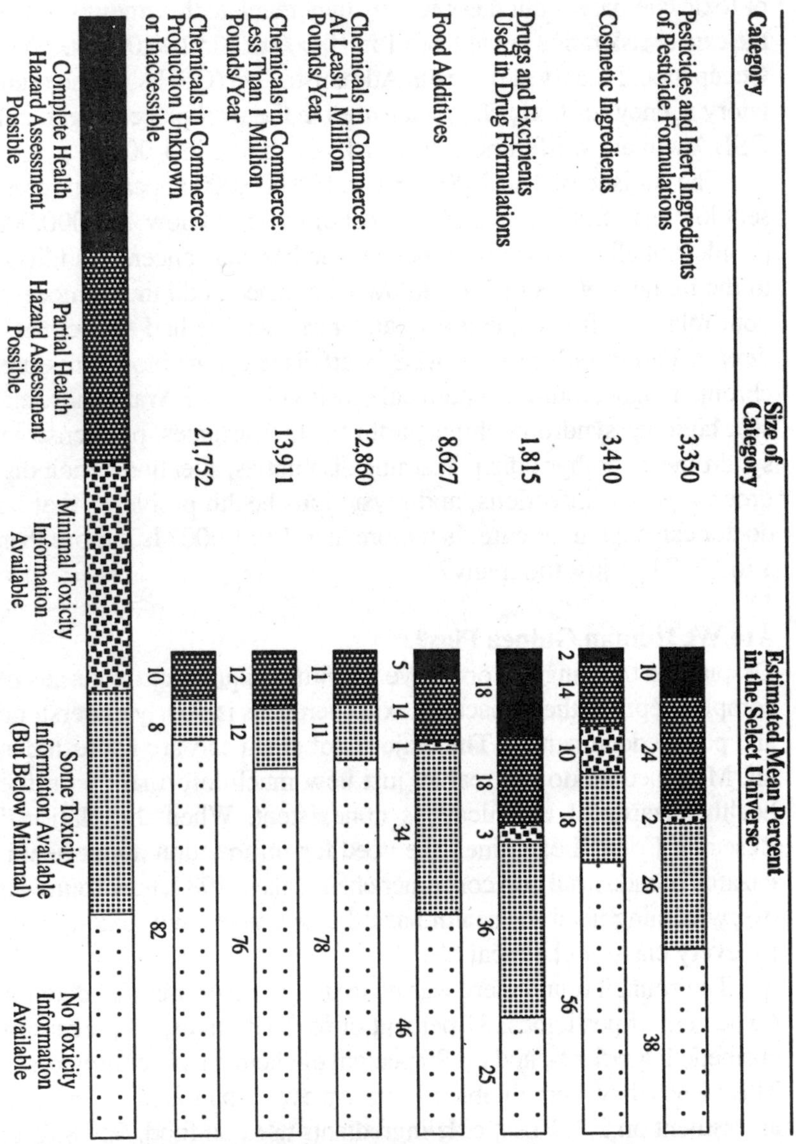

Category	Size of Category	Estimated Mean Percent in the Select Universe				
		Complete Health Hazard Assessment Possible	Partial Health Hazard Assessment Possible	Minimal Toxicity Information Available	Some Toxicity Information Available (But Below Minimal)	No Toxicity Information Available
Pesticides and Inert Ingredients of Pesticide Formulations	3,350	10	24	2	26	38
Cosmetic Ingredients	3,410	2	14	10	18	56
Drugs and Excipients Used in Drug Formulations	1,815	18	18	3	36	25
Food Additives	8,627	5	14	1	34	46
Chemicals in Commerce: At Least 1 Million Pounds/Year	12,860		11	11		78
Chemicals in Commerce: Less Than 1 Million Pounds/Year	13,911		12	12		76
Chemicals in Commerce: Production Unknown or Inaccessible	21,752		10	8		82

Ability to conduct health-hazard assessment of substances in seven categories on a select universe of chemicals

Figure 8.1

Reprinted with permission from TOXICITY TESTING STRATEGIES TO DETERMINE NEEDS AND PROPERTIES. © 1984 by the National Academy of Sciences. Courtesy of the National Academy Press, Washington, D.C.

When toxic chemicals are released without adequate neurotoxicity testing, human beings are the guinea pigs in experiments on safety. For example, we know that the soil fumigant DBCP can cause sterility because employees handling this product compared notes with one another.[37]

The 1988 EPA Pesticide Fact Sheet for the organophosphate pesticide malathion stated that "the existing data base of malathion is lacking chronic toxicity studies, an acceptable teratology study in rats [teratology means effects on the unborn], an acceptable reproduction study, mutagenicity studies, and a metabolism study. . . . Data gaps exist for environmental fate. . . . Data are needed before the Agency can assess the potential for malathion to contaminate groundwater." Data gaps were also found in the metabolism of malathion in plants and animals.[38]

With these overwhelming data gaps about malathion—the lack of information about long-term environmental effects, the impact of this neurotoxin on the next generation, and the health hazard of chronic exposure—it was awarded a provisional acceptable daily intake, which meant that it legally could be sold and used.

In 1989, malathion was sprayed by helicopters over most of the state of California to control the Mediterranean Fruit Fly. What are the long-term consequences of applying malathion over an entire state? Will there be an increase in birth defects? Will the IQ rates in the next generation decrease? Will Alzheimer's disease, Parkinson's disease, ALS, fatigue, headaches, and chronic illnesses increase? Will malathion accumulate in ground water? Why was this information not known before this neurotoxin was used so extensively?

Risk/Benefit Ratios
The risk assessments, which establish regulations on toxic chemicals, consider both health hazards and anticipated social benefits. A *risk/benefit ratio* is the term that expresses this concept of weighing the pros and cons of using a toxic chemical.

In pharmacology, scientists study the properties of drugs, both their healing properties and their side effects. The healing property of the drug is the benefit, while the side effects are the risk. You make a risk/benefit calculation for yourself when you take medications.

You know that a cold medicine can make you drowsy (a risk), but it can alleviate the symptoms of your cold (a benefit).

While a risk/benefit ratio is an important concept in pharmacology, it may not be appropriate when determining public policy. We don't receive a list of the potential side effects that come with the use of neurotoxins. With public policies, those who suffer the risks may not be the ones who receive the benefits.

So how do toxicologists make these decisions about acceptable risk? According to a basic textbook in toxicology, "Some of the factors considered in determining an acceptable risk are:

1. the need met by the substance
2. the adequacy and availability of alternative substances to meet the identified need
3. the anticipated extent of public use
4. employment considerations
5. economic considerations
6. effects on environmental quality
7. conservation of natural resources "[39]

Are our regulatory agencies more concerned about corporate risks than health risks? It's clear that health risks from neurotoxicity are severely underestimated. And what is the "benefit" in the risk/benefit ratio? Does it refer to social benefits or to corporate profits?

BUSINESS: PROFIT VERSUS PROTECTION

In business, a "cost/benefit ratio" calculates the risk that a company will be sued and lose a lawsuit against the amount of profit the company anticipates. For a company, "safety" (which is low risk) refers to safety from lawsuits.

Neurotoxic chemical production, sales, and distribution is a multibillion dollar industry. A company profiting from toxic chemical production will work to maintain its profit margin. When forced to produce risk assessments, the company representatives and scientists are likely to present the data in the most positive fashion. Sometimes companies present information that is misleading or grossly false.

Scientific Fraud

All scientific work is vulnerable to bias or overt manipulation. Research is based on the results of experiments. Experiments are like a series of questions. The results of an experiment depend on what question is being asked. If the question (the experimental design) is slightly altered, the answer (or results) will be different. A scientist can manipulate or falsify experimental data as easily as an accountant can manipulate or falsify financial records. This manipulation can be subtle or blatant.

Here's an example of subtle scientific manipulation. During safety testing for NutraSweet (aspartame), people were given a capsule containing dry, powdered NutraSweet and monitored for symptoms. This set-up seems innocuous, until you realize that aspartame (NutraSweet) is more toxic when it is in a liquid solution. The dry aspartame tested is not as toxic as the substance found in soft drinks.[40]

Journalist Michael Brown described a more obvious deception. He alleges that when Dow Chemical attempted to demonstrate to the EPA that the herbicide 2,4,5-T (Agent Orange) being used in Oregon did not increase birth defects and miscarriages, Dow researchers compared the incidence of birth defects and miscarriage to another town and found the rates to be similar. The other town was Midland, Michigan, where Dow Chemical is headquartered. The Midland plant is where this toxic herbicide was produced. Reportedly, the rates of birth abnormalities in Midland dramatically increased in the early 1970s, after large-scale production of Agent Orange. So the real evidence indicates that both of the towns exposed to 2,4,5-T had increased birth defects and miscarriages.[41]

In legitimate research, people who are exposed to a chemical (the experimental group) are compared with people who are not exposed (the control group). When both groups are exposed, you no longer have an experiment. When scientists knowingly expose both groups, they are engaging in fraud.

Reliable sources allege that industry-sponsored studies of MSG have been using aspartame (NutraSweet) as a flavoring agent in experiments since 1978. This means that one group (the control group) was exposed to NutraSweet, and the other group (the experimental group) was exposed to NutraSweet and MSG. The researchers then claimed that MSG did not cause headaches, because people in the control group also had headaches.[42] What these studies really demonstrate is that people exposed to both MSG and NutraSweet reported headaches.

Sometimes researchers engage in blatant fraud. In studies of NutraSweet, researchers have been accused of falsifying data, removing brain tumors in living animals so they wouldn't be counted at death, substituting healthy animals for sick ones, not reporting brain, uterus, and ovary tumors to the FDA, and failing to investigate instances of seizures in monkeys.[43]

∿

Toxic crime is a clean crime because the perpetrator may never have to encounter his victim. What's the likelihood that the person who manipulates an experiment will know the family whose baby is born deformed, or the senile grandparent, or the sick woman who visits doctor after doctor and gets no answers to her health problems?

The people who produce toxic products, legalize their use, and sell them can believe the false data that suggest these products are safe. Neurotoxins are big business.

CHAPTER NINE

CREATING A NONTOXIC HOME

How healthy is your home? If it's like the average home, it's more polluted than you think. The air inside a typical home is two to ten times more polluted than the outside air. Even in cities with high levels of air pollution, more contaminants can be detected inside homes than outside. The major sources of indoor air pollution are consumer products, such as bathroom deodorizers and moth repellents; personal activities, such as smoking; and building materials, such as paints and adhesives.[1]

This half of the book will help you recognize the sources of neurotoxins in your home—the place over which you have the most influence when it comes to neurotoxins—and tell you about less toxic or nontoxic alternatives. Each change you make brings some benefit.

Living in a nontoxic home gives your body a chance to recuperate and detoxify from outside exposures over which you have less or no control. A nontoxic home is one of the best defenses against neurotoxins in the outside air, in water supplies, at work, and in public places.

WHAT'S RIGHT FOR YOU?

As you think about making changes in your home, begin by thinking about your needs and goals to see which changes are most important to make now and which changes you want to make gradually.

Do you currently have health problems you think could be related to toxins? Does someone else in your family have health problems? Have you watched a relative suffer from cancer, Alzheimer's disease, or arthritis and want to avoid the same fate? Are you healthy and want to stay that way? Is contributing to a cleaner environment important to you?

If your health is affected, a top priority may be to make immediate changes in your home to reduce neurotoxins. If you suspect that your child is being affected by toxins, you're probably ready to take action right away.

Not everyone is ready to make immediate changes. You might be at a point where you're interested in making changes, but you want to do it gradually. Some people feel more comfortable with slow, consistent change, like using up the products in the cupboard and replacing them with nontoxic products when it's time to restock. Other people want to act before they lose interest or forget the material in this book. The following chapters speak to both approaches to change.

If you or someone in your home has health problems you suspect are related to neurotoxic chemicals, you may want to see what happens when you remove all the neurotoxins possible. You could begin by sealing and storing neurotoxic products in the garage for a couple of months while you use nontoxic products. If you begin to see improvement, you'll have evidence that neurotoxins play a role in your health problem.

Sometimes a daily record of symptoms, symptom severity, and the time the symptoms occur helps people find a pattern to their symptoms. Some see immediate improvement when neurotoxins are removed. Others still have symptoms, but they're less severe or less frequent. If you or someone in your home, particularly a child, has a health problem, you may want to keep notes about how often the symptoms occur and how severe they are so you won't miss gradual improvement. Sometimes removing neurotoxins has a preventive effect, so you can't know what would have happened if you were still using neurotoxins.

Once you know what your needs are, you'll want to evaluate the products you're using. You can calculate your own cost/benefit ratio by asking, Does this product bring any real benefit to my life? Some products that contain neurotoxins offer no benefits—scented toilet paper, for example. Using a fragrance-free, color-free product will be no loss to you. By making this small change, you're both reducing neurotoxins in your home and encouraging the manufacturer to sell a less toxic product. After all, manufacturers will sell whatever we're willing to buy.

What about chemical air fresheners? These are expensive consumer products that are so neurotoxic in laboratory tests that mice have actually died from being exposed to them.[2] That's the ultimate in neurotoxicity! Are air fresheners important to you? If not, remove them from your life and you'll save money and an unnecessary exposure to a neurotoxin. If air fresheners are important to you, you'll want to learn about nontoxic alternatives (chapter 10) so you can enjoy the benefit without paying the cost.

Some neurotoxic products bring genuine benefits. A car, for example, can improve the quality of your life. But until we're able to purchase propane, electric, or solar-powered cars, we need to be responsible about maintenance, disposal, and use of our automobiles.

Every change you make to reduce neurotoxic exposure will benefit you and may even benefit people you've never met. As we quit buying neurotoxic products, manufacturers will start producing the less toxic and nontoxic products we do buy. When manufacturers stop producing neurotoxic products, the workers who produce these products will stop being exposed to neurotoxic ingredients.

DETOXIFICATION

To be healthy in a toxic world, you need to reduce your intake of neurotoxins and increase your rate of detoxification. You can increase detoxification by a healthy lifestyle. Exercise, good nutrition, laughter, and loving relationships are all part of healthy human functioning. They allow the body to operate at peak efficiency.

The physical demands of exercise and the heat it generates in your body are thought to increase the rate at which fat cells release their load of stored toxins. It may be that we often feel better after using a sauna or a hot tub because the heat facilitates the detoxification process. Massage can also facilitate detoxification.

Some medical programs use exercise, sauna treatments, and massage to increase the rate of detoxification in people with chemical injuries. When someone with a chemical injury is exposed to heat, he may initially feel worse, because the stored toxins are released into the bloodstream. For this reason, these types of programs are medically supervised and vitamins, minerals, and supplements are added to facilitate the body's detoxification processes.

Good nutrition is designed to provide the body with necessary resources. But when someone is exposed to neurotoxins, supplementation can be important, because the body can get depleted of vitamin and mineral resources during detoxification. Certain vitamins and other nutrients, called antioxidants, help the body to detoxify more efficiently.

Vitamin C, vitamin E, vitamin A and beta carotene, the minerals selenium, magnesium, zinc, and the enzyme glutathione are widely recognized antioxidants. Because vitamins E and A accumulate in the body, no one should take too much of them. Too much of any mineral can be harmful. For example, selenium can have dangerous effects at doses above 450 mcg per day.

To use antioxidants and other supplements effectively, it's important to consult with a health professional who is properly trained in the use of vitamins, minerals, and other supplements. These are not innocuous substances, and it's important to use them in a safe and effective manner. Other herbs and vitamins are also recognized as having antioxidant properties.

༄

The following chapters contain information about where neurotoxic chemicals are found in everyday life and how to begin replacing toxic products with nontoxic products. Each chapter is a brief summary of information. These chapters do not begin to provide all of the information available; they are designed to highlight the most important information. If you want more details on a particular issue, consult one of the many books written on each topic.

It is not the intent of this book to market or endorse any particular product or product line but to provide practical information about how to get started using nontoxic products. The author has no financial ties to any of the products or companies mentioned. When specific brand names are used, it's because there is limited availability of other nontoxic alternatives or the author is not aware of other options.

When possible, information about how to obtain a safer product is mentioned without recommending a brand name. The information provided is limited by the author's experience, and you are encouraged to find other companies and other sources of nontoxic products.

Many people notice that when they replace their toxic products, they have more energy or their headaches disappear. There are other benefits as well. Nontoxic housecleaning products save money, and these basic ingredients can be used for more than one task, so they require less cabinet space.

∽

While many people are motivated to change to a nontoxic lifestyle because of health concerns, anyone can be motivated by a desire to reduce the amount of pollution in our world. A nontoxic lifestyle will benefit you, your family, your neighbors, your community, and the entire planet.

CHAPTER TEN

NONTOXIC HOUSECLEANING

Many people HATE housework. They feel fatigued and grouchy after cleaning. But this fatigue and irritability may be the result of neurotoxic chemical exposures, not the result of the physical work.

When you use neurotoxic chemicals in your home, the fumes remain long after you've used the product. Once the mist clears, the chemicals do not magically leave the room. Fumes from an oven cleaner do not disappear just because the oven is clean. And the better the insulation in your home, the more effectively the chemicals get trapped in the air. Everyone in the home, including pets, inhales these chemical fumes.

Drain openers, oven cleaners, toilet bowl cleaners, ammonia-based cleaners, chlorine bleach cleaners, and air fresheners can all contain hazardous chemicals. The containers of these products are a significant source of hazardous waste. The problem is significant enough to merit city and county government pamphlets about nontoxic cleaning alternatives to reduce the cost in hazardous waste disposal.

If the bottle is classified as hazardous waste, what about the product? The source of the hazardous waste could be sitting under your kitchen sink, and you may be using it.

Just because a household product is widely distributed doesn't mean it's safe. Brightly colored labels and advertising campaigns make these poisonous substances seem less dangerous than they are. In industry, there are some regulations about the use of toxic chemicals. In the home, there are no standards and no safety inspectors. Homemakers have no legal protection from high levels of neurotoxic chemicals. It's no wonder so many woman experience health problems.

Ask yourself these questions: Do these toxic products improve the quality of my life? Could I eliminate some of them without missing them? TV commercials promise us that magic bubbles, bald-headed genies, and dancing pine trees will help with our housework. These products certainly cost more money, but are they any more effective than their nontoxic counterparts? If not, we're paying for a fancy label and an expensive advertising blitz.

You don't need neurotoxic chemicals to keep your home clean. You can improve the air quality in your home by replacing toxic products with nontoxic products. It's a simple and effective way to reduce neurotoxins and maintain or improve your health and the health of your family. Nontoxic cleaning also contributes to the health of your community by reducing your city's hazardous waste. Perhaps the solution to hazardous waste disposal problems is to stop producing unnecessary hazardous waste!

NONTOXIC CLEANING

As you choose housecleaning products, you'll want to avoid neurotoxins like ammonia, chlorine bleach, petrochemicals, and "fragrance." Ammonia can be easily identified by its strong odor in products like glass cleaners, disinfectants, and all-purpose cleaners. It is a strong chemical that can cause "ammonia intoxication." In industry, there are standards to protect employees from an excess exposure to ammonia.[1]

Chlorine bleach is found in scouring powders, bathroom cleaners, and other bleach products. Byproducts of chlorine that can contaminate the air in your home include chloroform, trihalomethanes, and nonvolatile chlorinated hydrocarbons. Chlorine can also combine with other chemicals to produce new, more toxic substances. Many household products also contain petrochemicals.

When the term *fragrance* is listed as an ingredient, it can be any combination of some 5,000 to 6,000 fragrance chemicals.[2] Many of the chemicals used to produce fragrances are highly neurotoxic. They are an unnecessary source of neurotoxins in your home.

You can keep your home clean with the following basic, inexpensive, multi-purpose cleaning ingredients:

❖ Water
❖ Soap
❖ Nontoxic Scouring Powder
❖ Hydrogen Peroxide
❖ White Vinegar
❖ Borax
❖ Baking Soda

The single most effective cleaning agent available on our planet is nontoxic and free — water. Most housecleaning products are effective primarily because they're wet. It's the moisture that works, rather than the strong chemicals. For some jobs you'll want to add a nontoxic soap. Other jobs need a scouring agent, such as a scouring powder, baking soda, or borax. To cut grease, you can use vinegar. To sterilize, use hydrogen peroxide.

Vacuuming
Regular vacuuming will help keep your carpet clean. For a nontoxic carpet freshener, liberally apply baking soda and vacuum it up after about twenty minutes. Most commercial carpet fresheners use an ingredient like baking soda combined with a fragrance.

Mopping
The most effective ingredient for mopping is water and physical scrubbing. Depending on the type of cleaning you want to do, you can add different ingredients to the water. You may want to add a small amount of liquid soap, for example. If you want to cut grease or add shine to the floor, use a mixture of half water and half vinegar. If mopping with soap leaves your floor sticky, the vinegar/water mixture will remove the residue.

Dusting

To dust your home, you don't need to use a chemical spray; a cloth dampened with water works just as well. After all, the only reason the chemical sprays remove dust is that they're moist. A feather duster or dry cloth only stirs the dust up to then resettle. If you want to use a dry duster, find one that holds in the dust by using static electricity.

No chemical formula can reduce the number of times a home needs dusting. Electrostatic filters, which are discussed in chapter 18, physically trap airborne dust and reduce the amount of dusting needed.

Furniture Polish

You can make your own nontoxic furniture polish (wood polish) with three parts olive oil and 1 part white vinegar.[3] Another effective combination is one part lemon juice and two parts vegetable oil. If you purchase a commercial product, read the ingredients carefully. A vegetable oil base is nontoxic, whereas a petroleum oil base is neurotoxic. To avoid neurotoxins, also avoid an added "fragrance."

Glass Cleaner

A vinegar-based cleaner is as effective in cleaning glass as an ammonia-based cleaner, but it's nontoxic. You can make your own solution of half water and half vinegar in a spray bottle. This is the most economical option. You'll probably want to use white vinegar for cleaning, and there's no reason not to use the cheapest vinegar you can find. If you want to purchase a glass-cleaning product, there are commercial vinegar-based glass cleaners available in both regular grocery stores and in health food stores. Check the ingredients to be sure there's no ammonia or fragrance added.

All-Purpose Cleaners

Replace ammonia-based all-purpose cleaners with a vinegar-and-water solution. Vinegar is excellent at cutting grease. For a tougher job, use more vinegar and less water. For very greasy jobs, use straight vinegar or a concentrated vinegar.

You can also make all-purpose cleaning solutions with soap and water or borax and water. Add vinegar or lemon juice to cut grease. You can also purchase nontoxic all-purpose cleaners at health food stores.

Tile and Porcelain

To clean tile, countertops, sinks, tubs, and toilets, use a nontoxic scouring powder. The best nontoxic commercial scouring powder I'm aware of is Bon Ami Kitchen and Bath Cleanser. Unlike other commercial scouring powders, it doesn't contain chlorine bleach and will not scratch most surfaces. It's widely available in regular grocery stores. You can also use baking soda or borax for scouring. Baking soda is very economical for cleaning tubs and toilets.

Disinfectants

It's not necessary to use an ammonia or chlorine bleach solution to kill germs on sinks and toilets. Regular cleaning prevents germs and other unhealthy organisms from multiplying. By keeping surfaces dry, you will create an environment in which bacteria, mildew, and mold cannot survive.[4]

Disinfectant chemical sprays are a completely unnecessary product that may or may not kill germs, but they will pollute the air in your home. These neurotoxic chemicals do not protect your family from illness. In fact, they can reduce your ability to fight off illness because they place an extra burden on the body to detoxify from the chemical assault. To top it off, these strong cleaning solutions do not eliminate all the germs; they only kill the germs they actually touch.

Rather than immerse your entire bathroom in a bleach solution, you can make your own effective, nontoxic cleaning solutions. A combination of borax (½ cup) in hot water (one gallon) is an effective germ killer.[5] Another alternative is to rinse a sink, shower, or toilet with inexpensive hydrogen peroxide, especially if a family member is ill.

If a stronger disinfectant is needed, Zephiran Chloride produced by Winthrop Pharmaceuticals in New York can be ordered by your pharmacist. Dilute this product according to the instructions.

Mold and Mildew

The best treatment for mold and mildew is borax. Borax is a naturally occurring mineral composed of sodium, boron, oxygen, and water.

The most recognized brand name is 20-Mule Team Borax. You can remove visible mold with a solution of borax and water or a solution of vinegar and water. To prevent future mold growth, sponge on a solution of borax and water to bathroom or shower walls and leave it to dry. To prevent mold growth under a kitchen or bathroom sink, sprinkle dry borax in the cabinet.

Mold can't survive in warm, dry places. Heat and light will eliminate it. A hand-held hair dryer or heater can get rid of moisture from an area and prevent the climate that mold requires to grow.[6]

Soap

One of the most effective cleaning agents is plain soap. Try to find a soap that doesn't contain fragrances or other petrochemicals. There are several good cleaning soaps sold through home-distribution product lines. Some of these companies have recently added fragrance to their products. If the fragrance is from a natural source, it would not be neurotoxic, but this can be difficult to verify. The Neo-Life home distribution network continues to sell fragrance-free Green Soap and Rugged Red.

Some of the brands of nontoxic dishwashing soaps, which are carried by health food stores and can be used as an all-purpose cleaner, include Granny's Old Fashioned Products, Allen's Naturally, and Ecover. For dishes, you can add 20-Mule Team Borax to dishwater or a dishwasher to prevent water spots. Dishwasher detergents are available from Allen's Naturally and Ecover.

Oven Cleaners

If you don't want to clean your oven very often, just make sure that food doesn't get spilled in it. Use a larger pan when cooking, place a cookie sheet underneath to catch drips, or clean a spill before it has hardened.

When you have to clean your oven, there are simple, nontoxic alternatives to chemical oven cleaners. You can mix baking soda with just enough water to form a paste, apply it to the oven, and leave it to dry for twenty minutes. When you scrub it off, most of the grime will come off. You can use a little scouring powder to remove any remaining grime. For a super dirty job, apply the baking soda paste twice. Another nontoxic solution is two tablespoons of liquid soap and two teaspoons of borax in warm water. After it dries for about twenty minutes, scrub it off with steel wool and scouring powder.[7]

You may notice a big difference in how you feel after using these completely safe solutions compared to how you feel after using a highly toxic chemical oven cleaner. You'll probably be less tired, even if you had to scrub a little bit harder.

Drain Cleaners

Drain cleaners that contain lye are a dangerous and unnecessary household product. You can pour boiling water down the drain to prevent clogs or remedy a slow-draining sink. You may need to remove hair to prevent clogs in a shower drain. If you have a clogged drain, a combination of a handful of baking soda and ½ cup of white vinegar will cause a chemical reaction to dislodge the clog. If you've ever combined vinegar and baking soda in a school science project, you know how they react. Cover the drain tightly for a couple of minutes and then follow with hot water. You can also find some natural products that use enzymes or other digestive organisms to unclog drains.[8]

Air Fresheners

Air fresheners are a major source of indoor air pollution. Solid dispensers and products you plug in continually re-infest a room with neurotoxic substances. Dr. Rosalind Anderson (who did studies on carpet samples) has recently begun testing the effects of air fresheners on mice. She's finding that mice exposed to fumes from solid air fresheners have severe neurotoxic reactions, and in some cases are dying as a result of the neurotoxic fumes.[9]

Commercial air fresheners exist as a result of successful advertising campaigns. If there's a foul odor in your home, spraying a chemical to mask it only adds a toxic chemical to the source of the stench. The only way to effectively remove odors is to keep your home clean, open the windows, and remove garbage or other sources of odor. To get that "outdoor, garden-fresh smell," open the window!

A bowl of baking soda can absorb odors in a room, just as it does in the refrigerator. A bowl of white vinegar can also be placed in a room to absorb odors. You can purchase a product called a Molecular Adsorber which pulls odors, chemicals, and molds out of the air by attracting water molecules into its very dry contents (see appendix A). These options actually eliminate odors, rather than cover them with a perfume. If the odor is from a garbage can, clean it and sprinkle borax in the bottom. If the odor comes from cigarette smoke, smoke outside (and work on quitting). If the odor is from a cat box, you can add baking soda to the cat litter, clean the box more often, or use a Molecular Adsorber next to the box.

If you like air fresheners, potpourri, or candles because of their fragrance, find a natural source, such as fragrant herbs in boiling water. You can make a natural potpourri by using herbs, natural essential oils (see chapter 12), or cedar shavings. Commercial air fresheners that use natural sources of fragrances are also available at health food stores.

A NATURAL CLEAN

I once walked into a hotel lobby and watched a staff member sitting in the corner, occasionally spraying a chemical cleaner into the air instead of using it to clean. There was a strong smell, but nothing was clean. The dust was still on the tables and the smudges were still on the glass.

It's important to know the difference between a clean home and the odor of bleach or ammonia in cleaning products. The occasional use of highly toxic cleaners is not a substitute for regular cleaning. It takes consistent cleaning and early intervention, like wiping a spill before it dries or drying out a cabinet before it mildews. This is the cleanest, easiest, and least toxic option.

Although some toxic cleaning products sometimes reduce the amount of effort required in scrubbing, exercising your muscles may be less fatiguing than inhaling the fumes of neurotoxic chemicals.

In addition to providing a healthier home and reducing pollutants, nontoxic cleaning saves money, requires less cabinet space, and prevents accidental poisoning in children.

Advertisers are experts at making us feel insecure about ourselves if we don't purchase their products. But these products cost too much in terms of fatigue, cancer, hazardous waste dumps, and accidental poisonings.

CHAPTER ELEVEN

NONTOXIC PEST CONTROL

There's something seductive about eliminating an annoying problem like bugs by simply pushing a button on a can of bug spray. It's kind of like shooting the bad guys in an old Western movie.

The fact that neurotoxic pesticides are sold in our grocery stores as sprays and bombs would seem to indicate they're safe to use in our homes. But the majority of these products contain organophosphate or carbamate pesticides. These are highly toxic substances which are neurotoxic to humans as well as to insects.

ORGANOPHOSPHATE PESTICIDES

Organophosphate pesticides are among the most poisonous substances used in pest control. They are rapidly metabolized by the body, and a person can die within five minutes when overexposed.[1] Hallucinations, depression, and psychosis have been caused by organophosphate pesticide exposures. Mild cases of poisoning have caused lapses of attention or judgment that led to accidents, particularly for crop duster pilots.[2] Organophosphate poisoning can mimic psychosis, chronic fatigue, digestive disorders, and upper respiratory infection.[3]

Chronic poisoning can cause headeache, weakness, decline in memory, quick fatigue, disturbed sleep, loss of appetite, and disorientation.[4] Does this list of symptoms sound familiar? These are the symptoms of an injured nervous system (see chapter 2).

There are numerous reports of long-term impairment following organophosphate poisoning. The long-term consequences on mental functioning can include: impaired vigilance and reduced concentration, slowed information processing and rate of response, memory problems, language disturbances, depression, anxiety, and irritability.[5] These symptoms could destroy the career of an adult. A child demonstrating these deficits in school would be at a permanent disadvantage.

When you know the history of organophosphate pesticides, you will understand why they are so hazardous to humans. They're the direct descendants of "nerve gas" developed for chemical warfare. Chemical weapons were one of the first weapons of mass destruction, and after the atrocities of World War I, over 140 countries signed the Geneva Protocol in 1925 to prohibit the use of these poisonous gases in future wars. Following this ban, chemists found other ways to utilize the deadly technology. Nerve gas began to be used to destroy other life forms.

Chemical weapons earned the name "nerve gas" because they interfere with the communication of the central nervous system by destroying the enzyme acetylcholinesterase. Each time the nervous system communicates to the muscles, the neurotransmitter acetylcholine is released. After this release, acetylcholinesterase removes the leftover acetylcholine so the next communication between nerve cells can occur. Nerve gas kills by destroying acetylcholinesterase.

If you read the warning label on the side of a can of bug spray, it may tell you to use atropine in case of accidental poisoning. Atropine is the treatment of choice for acute pesticide poisoning. Atropine has only one other use. It is the antidote to exposure during chemical warfare. When American soldiers are at war, they carry an injection of atropine.

The following chart details some of the organophosphate pesticides:

A PARTIAL LISTING OF ORGANOPHOSPHATE PESTICIDES[6]

PESTICIDE	TRADE NAMES	USES
Diazinon	Spectracide, Diazitol, Neocidol, Nucidol, Basudin, Dipofene	Household insects, soil insects, foliage insects, agricultural insects
Chlorpyrifos	Dursban, Lorsban	Mosquitoes, flies, household insects, foliage crop pests, aquatic larvae
Malathion	Malathion, Malathon Chemathion, Cythion, Emmaton, Karbophos, Malaspray, Malathiozol, Malathiozoo	Mosquitoes, flies, Mediterranean fruit fly, household pests, human lice, animal parasites
Parathion	Alkron, Alleron, Aphamite, Bladan, Etilon, Folidol, Fosferno, Niram, Paraphos, Rhodiatox	Agricultural, nursery, greenhouse use, fly control
Parathion-methyl	Bladan M, Dalf, Folidol-M, Metacide, Metron, Nitrox	Similar to parathion
Dichlorvos	De-Pester Insect Strip, Oko, Kill-Fly Resin Strip, Mafu, No-Pest Strip, Phoracide, Nuvan, Crossman's Fly-Cake, Dedevap, Task Canogard, Estrosol, Hercol, Herkol, Lethalaire, Misect, Phosvit, Vapona, Vaponicide, Vaporette Bar, Nogos, Atgard, Dichlorman, Equigard	Flies, horseflies, mosquitoes, fleas, used in restaurants, food-handling businesses, homes, pet flea collars, animal shelters, airplanes, greenhouses, warehouses, tobacco
TEPP (tetraethyl pyrophosphate)	Kilmite, Killex, Bladan, Fosnex, Gy-Tet 40, HETP, Hexaethyltetraphos-phate, Lethalaire, Teep, Licophosphate, Nifos T, Pyfos, Phro-Phos, Tetradusto 100, Tetron, Tetraspa, Vapotone	Aphids, spiders, mites, mealy bugs, leafhoppers, thrips

PESTICIDE	TRADE NAMES	USES
Dialifos	Torak	Insects and mites common to apples, citrus, grapes, nut trees, potatoes, vegetables
Trichlorfon	Anthon, Dipterex, Dylox, Dyrex, Foschlor, Neguvon, Masoten, Proxol, Tugon	Flies, roaches, worms and other parasites in animals
Schradan	Pestox III, Pestox 3, Sytam	Mites, sap-feeding insects
Temephos	Abat, Abate, Abathion, Biothion, Bithion, Nimitex, Swebate	Larvae of mosquitoes, midges, flies and moths, human body lice, used on crops
Phenthoate	Cidial, Elsan, Papthion, PAP, Tanone, Tsidial	Moths, leafhoppers, aphids, mosquito larvae and adults
Carbophenothion	Acarithion, Garrathion, Trithion	Aphids, mites, ticks, used as a dormant spray for overwintering mites, aphids and scale insects due to long residual action
Naled	Bromex, Dibrom	Mites, ticks, adult mosquitoes, and other insects, used on plants under glass and in mushroom houses
Chlorfenvinphos	Birlane, Dermaton, Sapecron, Supona	Foliage and soil, mites on pets
Phosalone	Rubitox, Zolone	Mites, ticks, insects, used on fruit trees, market garden crops, cotton, potatoes
Dichlofenthion	Bromex, Hexa-nema, V-C 13, Mobilawn, Nemacide	Worms, parasites, used as a soil insecticide
Dioxathion	Co-Nav, Delnav, Kavadel, Navadel	Citrus mites, ticks and other external pests on livestock
Dimefox	Hanane, Pestox IV, S-14	Aphids, spiders, red spider mites on hops, and other insects

PESTICIDE	TRADE NAMES	USES
Mipafox	Isopestox, Pestox 15, Pestox XV	Unspecified
Dicapthon	Dicaptan, Isomeric Clorthio, Isomer of Clorthion	Aphids and other insects
Dimethoate	Cygon, De-Fend, Dimetate Ferkethion, Fostion MM, Perfekthion, Rogor, Roxion	Mites, ticks, and other insects
Endothion	Endocide	Aphids, sap-feeding insects and mites in orchards, fields, and market garden crops
Fenthion	Baycid, Baytex, Entex Lebaycid, Mercaptophos, Queletox, Spotton, Tiguvon	Fruit flies, leafhoppers, cereal bugs
Methidathion	Supracide, Ultracide, Ustracide	Scale insects, leaf eaters, mites
Mevinphos	Phosdrin	Unspecified
Dicrotophos	Bidrin, Carbicron, Ektafos	Unspecified
Demeton	Systox	Mites, sap-feeding insects
Demeton-methyl	Metasystox, Meta-isosystox	Mites, ticks, and other insects, used on cotton
Oxydemeton-methyl	Metasystox R	Mites, sucking insects

A PARTIAL LISTING OF CARBAMATE PESTICIDES[7]

PESTICIDE	TRADE NAMES	USES
Carbaryl	Carbacide, Carpolin, Denopton Karbatox, Mervin, Sevinox, Sevin	Contact insecticide (unspecified)
Aldicarb	Temik	Spiders, mites, ticks, and other insects
Propoxur	Baygon, Blattanex, Invisi-Gard, Sendra, Sendran, Undene, Suncide, Tendex, Unden	Mosquitoes, used for rapid "knock down" of agricultural and household pests

PESTICIDE	TRADE NAMES	USES
Carbofuran	Furadan, Yaltox	Systemic and contact insecticide (unspecified)
Dioxacarb	Elecron, Elocron, Famid Flocron, Gamid	Aphids, cockroaches, household pests, pests in stored products, used for rapid "knockdown" action
Landrin	Landrin	Corn
Methomyl	Lannate, Nudrin	Unspecified
Mexacarbate	Zectran, Mexacarbate	Mites, ticks, snails, worms
Oxamyl	Vydate	Aphids, flea beetles, worms
Promecarb	Carbamult, Minacide	Beetles, moths

A PARTIAL LISTING OF CHLORINATED HYDROCARBON PESTICIDES[8]

PESTICIDE	TRADE NAMES	USES
DDT (dichlorodiphenyl-trichloroethane)	Anofex, Cesarex Dinocide, Neocidol, Neocid, Gesarol, Gyron, Guesapon, Guesarol, Ixodex, Zerdane	Flies, mosquitoes, forest pests and agricultural pests, now banned in U.S.
Ethylan	Perthane	Leafhoppers, moths, larvae, and carpet beetles
Methoxychlor	Marlate	Agricultural insects
BHC (benzene hexachloride)	BHC, Lindane, 666, Tri-6, Agrocide, Benexane, Ben-Hex, Borer-Tox, Ambrocide Kwell, Quellada, Aparasin, Lindatox, Borekil, Aphtiria,Gammexane, Gexane, Gamasan, Ambrocide, Jacutin, Lorexane, Streunex, gamma-BHC, Benesan	Grasshoppers, soil pests, treating seeds, household insects, and livestock
Chlordane	Chlordane, Belt, Corodane, Niran, Octachlor, Octa-Klor, Synklor, Toxichlor	Termites, agricultural pests

PESTICIDE	TRADE NAMES	USES
Heptachlor	Drinox, Heptagran, Heptamul	Termites, was used for agriculture, but EPA limited usage in 1975
Aldrin (breaks down into dieldrin in the body)	Aldrex, Octalene, Toxadrin	Vegetable and fruit pests, field and forage pests
Dieldrin	Alvit, Octalox, Panoram, Quintox	Agricultural fields, soil treatments, sprayed in homes in tropical countries
Endosulfan	Thiodan, Beosit, Cyclodan, Malix, Thifor, Thimul	Agricultural pests
Mirex	Mirex	Fire ants
Chlordecone	Kepone	Leaf-eating insects and fly larvae
Toxaphene	Toxaphene, Toxadust, Agricide Maggot Killer, Alltox, Chem-Phene Estonox, Geniphene, Gyphene, Phenacide, Phenatox, Toxakil, Toxaspra	Cotton pests, agricultural animals, mites, vegetable pests

Malathion and diazinon are particularly subject to chemical changes during storage.[9] This means the chemical that is actually applied could be many times more toxic than the chemical tested and licensed. Both of these neurotoxins are widely used.

It's ironic when you consider there's a world-wide treaty banning the use of organophosphate compounds as a weapon of war, yet our city and state governments can legally use organophosphate pesticides in their war on insects.

Parathion has the distinction of causing more cropworker poisonings in the U.S. than any other pesticide. Parathion-contaminated food and clothing have caused hundreds of deaths. Many children have died from being treated for head lice with parathion.[10]

Dialifos was used in the 1980s in agriculture to control insects and mites in apples, citrus, grapes, nut trees, potatoes, and vegetables. Dialifos is chemically related to thalidomide, the drug which caused children to be born with deformed arms and legs. The potential of dialifos to cause birth defects was not known. The teratology (impact of the chemical on developing babies) of this compound has not been adequately studied.[11]

CARBAMATE PESTICIDES

The carbamate pesticides are another major class of neurotoxic pesticides that inhibit acetylcholinesterase. Carbamates that do not alter acetylcholinesterase are used as herbicides or fungicides.[12] Some of the pesticides in this class of neurotoxins are listed on pages 108-109.

Carbamates are considered to be less toxic than the organophosphate pesticides. However, the changes in acetylcholinesterase caused by carbamate poisoning are difficult to measure using current techniques. As a result, the toxicity of these compounds may be seriously underestimated.[13] In practical terms, the symptoms and treatment of carbamate poisoning are similar to those of the organophosphates.

CHLORINATED HYDROCARBON PESTICIDES

The third major category of neurotoxic pesticides is the chlorinated hydrocarbon pesticides, which are also known as organochlorine pesticides. This group of pesticides includes those listed in the chart on pages 109-110.

The chlorinated hydrocarbon pesticides were formulated to be longer lasting and less acutely lethal than the organophosphate pesticides. They certainly are long-lasting. One of the chlorinated pesticides, chlordane, remains toxic after twenty years![14] Chlordane has been applied to over 30 million homes in the U.S. to prevent termites. In 1982 the National Research Council stated that they "could not determine a level of exposure to the [cyclodiene] termiticides below which there would be no biologic effects."[15]

When chlordane is applied underneath a home, it contaminates the air inside the home. In a study of over forty homes treated with chlordane and heptachlor, some level of the toxic chemical was measured in the air of every home tested. The state of New York has permanently banned the use of chlordane because of the human and environmental hazard.

In 1987, the Velsicol company made an agreement with the EPA that they would not sell chlordane in the U.S., but they could still produce and export it. In 1988, the EPA allowed them to apply chlordane to another 150 homes to monitor the air levels.[16] Chlordane is a dangerous chemical that should not be used, even if the ban is lifted.

Another chlorinated hydrocarbon banned for use in the United States is DDT. It continues to be produced and exported around the world. When farmers in other countries are unable to read the application instructions, they can over-apply it to a severe degree. So we haven't really banned DDT from use in the United States, since DDT-contaminated food is regularly imported into the U.S. and sold in our supermarkets.[17] DDT continues to be measured in human breast milk.

NON-NEUROTOXIC PEST CONTROL

The use of neurotoxic pesticides in homes, yards, and offices is extensive. The average person is exposed to 1.1 pounds of active pesticide ingredients each year from nonagricultural sources.[18]

Pesticides are created to be neurotoxic to living creatures. Their sole purpose is to destroy the central nervous system of a bug. Yet a neurotoxin does not distinguish between the living cells of an insect and the living cells of a human. Bugs are more vulnerable because of their small size. But after the bugs in your home are killed, who's the next smallest in size? Your pet? Your child? Yourself?

Pest control should not have to be deadly to all forms of life. The effectiveness of non-neurotoxic pest control is comparable in getting rid of bugs while protecting the health of animals and humans.While neurotoxic pest control is like shooting the bad guys, non-neurotoxic pest control is more like tracking down big game and setting an effective trap.

The following pages will suggest nontoxic alternatives for controlling common pests around your home.

Roaches

The first step in non-neurotoxic pest control is prevention. Since roaches and ants are attracted to food stuck on cabinets and left on dirty dishes, cleanliness is the best way to prevent infestations. Keeping the kitchen clean and sealing food will make your home less interesting to bugs.

Roaches are also attracted to clutter, such as paper bags or a pile of old newspapers. They need to have things touching them in order to mate. Keeping the areas between kitchen cabinets, under stairs, and in the attic clear of clutter can interfere with roach romance. Since roaches are active when it's dark, you're most likely to see them when you enter a dark kitchen and flip on the light. At the first sign of roaches, it's time for intervention.

The most effective substance to use against roaches is boric acid, which is a stomach poison, not a neurotoxin. Boric acid is so effective that even companies that produce highly toxic pest control products may offer a boric acid product. It is sold as a powder and is available in most hardware stores and many grocery stores under various brand names, such as Roach Pruf and Roach Ridd. According to a former EPA entomologist, William Curry, boric acid has been found to be 90 percent effective in killing roaches, whereas dangerous neurotoxic pesticides are only 60 percent effective.[19] Boric acid will continue to kill roaches as long as it is kept dry. It needs to be lightly sprinkled or poofed with a bulb duster or plastic squeeze bottle to create a thin layer of powder for the roaches to walk on.

Boric acid will be poisonous to children or pets if they ingest a large quantity of it, so apply it in places where children or pets can't reach it. It should be applied in cracks and crevices where it can remain effective for years. When a roach walks through boric acid, the powder sticks to its feet and antennae. The roach is poisoned when it cleans its feet and ingests the boric acid.

Bait traps or bug motels that kill the roach by trapping it with a sticky glue are another good alternative, but you want to be sure a neurotoxic pesticide hasn't been added.

Ants

Boric acid is also effective in killing ants. Ants move in a predictable pattern and follow a trail. Find where the trail enters your home and you may be able to physically seal off the entryway; or put boric acid in front of the hole to prevent entry. Wipe up the current trail of ants with a wet, soapy paper towel or cloth. Sometimes you can get rid of a mild invasion of ants simply by spraying the trail with biodegradable soap. You can also sprinkle boric acid along the trail so the ants walk through the poison.

To create a poisonous bait, mix boric acid into a few drops of either a vegetable oil or sweetened jelly placed on a disposable paper plate. Place a light powdering of boric acid around the poisoned bait so the ants also have to walk through it. Oil-seeking ants will be attracted to the vegetable oil, and sugar-seeking ants will be attracted to the jelly. If you put down the poisoned oil or jelly, be prepared for a swarm of ants to come eat the poison. Usually there's a swarm of ants for a couple of days, which dwindles as the colony is destroyed. Ants take the poison back to their home base. When they die, the other ants eat them, and this poisons the colony. It's usually best to put the poison near the entry place or even outside so the ants are not tracking through your home. Be sure the poisoned bait is out of reach of children or pets.

Another poisoned bait recipe is to mix three cups of water with one cup of sugar and four teaspoons of boric acid. Pour the solution into jelly jars with cotton balls. To protect children and pets, you can poke holes in the jar lids and place the lids back on the jar. You can smear some of the solution on the outside of the jar. Place the jars in a location where you can tolerate the incoming ants.[20]

Dry boric acid powder can also be used outside on the anthill or at the outside entry point into your home. When it gets wet, it loses effectiveness, so you may need to reapply it regularly. You should see results within a few days. Another way to attack an anthill is to pour boiling water or hot paraffin down the nest entrance, but be careful to protect your feet from a swarm of ants.

Your goal is not to destroy all ants. The common house ant is a natural enemy of termites, so nonbiting ants outside are very beneficial. If you have any cracks around the house, seal them up to help keep your home ant-free while keeping these natural termite killers in your yard. Mint planted close around the house is a natural ant repellent.

Spiders
Neurotoxic pesticides do not work with spiders; the "squish method" does. Manually crushing the spider and removing the web

is the most effective method for combatting them.

Spiders are less likely to inhabit a clean house. Remove any cobwebs along the edges of the ceiling or in corners. Outdoor spiders should usually be left alone, except for poisonous black widows or brown recluses. Spiders serve a useful purpose by trapping and killing many other annoying insects.

Moths

Mothballs produce harmful fumes that can permeate an entire home. They should never be used. In our grandparents' generation, woolens were stored in cedar chests to prevent moth damage. Cedar blocks placed in clean fabrics are an alternative to mothballs. They are available in many hardware and storage specialty stores.

The moths you see are not the moths that damage fabrics. It's the larva of the clothes moth which feasts on woolens and other fabrics, and this moth is usually too small to notice. Moth eggs can be killed by laying the fabric in the sun or running it through a warm clothes dryer. They can also be killed by placing the fabric in the freezer for several days. The larvae are attracted to soiled fabrics, especially food-stained fabrics, so keeping items clean will prevent an infestation. Washing fabrics destroys all forms of these moths. After carefully washing linens or clothes (or using a heat or freezing treatment), store them in an airtight container to protect from moths.[21]

Fleas

Many people bomb their homes with pesticides to get rid of fleas. Flea bombs and other insect bombs are highly dangerous to humans and animals and should never be used. Again, boric acid is a very effective treatment. In fact, there are companies in many cities that specialize in treating homes with a combination of boric acid and carpet freshener, which they apply to the carpet and then vacuum up. The company should guarantee the treatment for a year, and if the fleas return, the company should return for free.

It's important to treat for fleas early in the infestation, because a full-blown infestation is more difficult to combat than a few wayward pests. A mild infestation of fleas can even be combatted with the vacuum cleaner. A thorough vacuuming will remove most of the fleas and their eggs. Be sure to dispose of the vacuum bag in an outside trash can or the larvae in the bag will re-infest your home. Vacuum the house daily if you have an infestation and weekly to prevent a flea problem.

For a moderate to severe infestation, you can bake fleas out of your home by turning up the heat to the highest setting and leaving the house for the day. In some parts of the country, this can be achieved in the summertime by simply turning off the air-conditioning.

The easiest way to combat fleas in your home is not to have an animal in the house. But since this isn't always desirable, here are some other options. For cat owners, having the cat live exclusively indoors or outdoors will prevent it from carrying outdoor fleas into the home. For dog owners, keeping the dog outdoors in the summertime, during the height of the flea season, will make it easier to keep fleas out of the house.

If you have an indoor animal, the fleas will accumulate where the animal sleeps, so establish a consistent sleeping place with bedding that is easy to wash. The bedding should be washed weekly when the house is being vacuumed. The area underneath bedding can be dusted with a natural repellent such as diatomaceaous earth (a powder made from fossilized sea plankton, which is razor sharp to bugs) or cedar shavings.

To prevent fleas from attacking your pet, groom your pet daily with a fine-toothed flea comb during the height of the season, and less often during the year. The comb will remove fleas and their eggs. Dip the comb in a bucket of soapy water every few strokes to drown the fleas. If you don't get any fleas after a thorough combing, you can comb your pet less frequently. Another effective way to kill fleas is to bathe your pet in soap and water. If you begin bathing your pet from the time it is very young, it will probably cooperate with the bathing process. A healthy pet is better able to resist flea attacks.

The use of neurotoxic pesticides on a pet is cruel to the animal and dangerous to the people living with the pet. Cats, dogs, and humans are not able to develop resistance to neurotoxic pesticides, even though fleas are. Flea treatments—neurotoxic flea bombs, shampoos, and collars—are the primary cause of poisoning in animals. Daily use of a carbamate pesticide can kill your pet. In one case, both a cat and his owner, a fifty-year-old professor of medicine, became aggressive after using a carbamate pesticide on the cat. The cat began killing small animals, and the professor was in a state of rage.[22] If both a person and a pet are ill in your home, it would be worth considering whether a neurotoxic chemical is involved.

In addition to bathing or combing your pet, vacuuming your house, and using a boric acid treatment, there are a variety of natural flea repellents. These repellents do not kill the fleas, but they make the flea more likely to go elsewhere. A variety of herbal collars are available at pet stores and health food stores. The most frequently used natural repellents include pennyroyal oil, eucalyptus oil, citronella oil, and tea tree oil. Another flea repellent is natural pyrethrins, which are derived from chrysanthemums.

The oil in citrus peels also repels fleas and other insects. You can make an anti-flea lotion by cutting four lemons in eighths, covering them with water, and bringing the mixture to a boil. Simmer for forty-five minutes, then cool and strain the liquid. Store the solution in a glass container. To use on your pet, wet the animal thoroughly with the solution and brush the wet fur so the lemon juice and the oil from the peel penetrate to the skin. After drying the animal, brush again.[23]

Several yard plants are thought to repel fleas. In the South, wax myrtle has been planted near the foundation of homes to repel fleas, and the herb pennyroyal can be planted around the outside of the home and around the lawn or garden.[24]

Lice

Neurotoxic pesticides successfully kill lice. Unfortunately, they can also kill people. Parathion and lindane are heavy-duty pesticides which have been used to treat head lice and have resulted in the death of children. Neurotoxic chemicals are able to penetrate skin and enter directly into the bloodstream. A neurotoxin in a shampoo easily penetrates the skin of the scalp and enters the bloodstream in the brain. No louse is worth permanent neurotoxic poisoning in a child.

Some shampoos use pyrethrins as the active ingredient (natural pyrethrums are derived from chrysanthemums). However, the inactive ingredients used with the pyrethrum can be a petroleum distillate or a solvent. You will not know which inactive ingredients are used, because neurotoxins can be legally hidden under the term *inert ingredient*. In English, the word *inert* means "deficient in active properties or lacking the power to move." It implies an inactive, unimportant additive. In the language of pesticides, inert means "these are the ingredients that will not be revealed."

Sometimes the inert ingredients are actually more toxic than the pesticide listed as the active ingredient. Solvents, such as xylene, an industrial toxin, are often used as an inert ingredient. Sometimes a chlorinated hydrocarbon pesticide is used as an "inert" ingredient![25] This means that a dangerous, long-lasting pesticide can be included in a product and the consumer doesn't have to be informed of its presence.

Using unknown chemicals on a child's scalp is an enormous risk. Fortunately, lice have a natural enemy in the coconut. Coconut oil contains dodecyl alcohol, which is deadly to adult lice. Coconut oil is often listed as "sodium lauryl sulfate" on a shampoo bottle. If there's an outbreak of lice at school, use coconut oil shampoo on your child preventively, and teach your child not to share a comb or brush with others.

If someone has a full-scale infestation of lice, it can be treated by thoroughly shampooing with a coconut-based shampoo, rinsing, lathering up the hair again, and leaving the soap in the hair with a towel tied around it for thirty minutes. Comb the soapy hair to remove tangles, then use a nit-removing comb to remove the eggs. If the hair dries, add water. Clean the comb repeatedly during this process. Afterwards, boil the comb, brush, and towels. After combing, rinse and wash again. Then inspect the hair for any other nits (eggs).

Another alternative is to warm a coconut oil solution (not too hot), pour it on the child's head at bedtime, and gently massage it into the hair. Cover the child's head with a cotton knit cap that ties under the chin. In the morning, wash twice with shampoo and comb carefully to remove eggs. Repeat weekly until the infestation is gone.

If one person in a family has contracted head lice, the whole family will need to shampoo daily with the coconut oil shampoo and comb dry hair, checking for lice. Wash pillow cases, sheets, and clothes frequently, vacuum upholstered furniture, and run pillows and blankets through the dryer to help prevent others from attracting lice. As with all pest control, early detection makes the problem easier to combat.[26]

Rats and Mice

One time-tested way to repel rodents is having a cat. With mice, even the odor of a kitten may encourage them to leave. Most people use mechanical traps with a food bait. Peanut butter is a good choice. Sprinkle boric acid powder around the trap so that any fleas or mites exiting the rodent are also killed.

Another alternative is to create non-neurotoxic rodent poisons. Mix one part plaster of Paris with one part flour, and season it with sugar or cocoa powder. Sprinkle it where rats and mice will find it.[27] Or cover a small pile of cement powder with flour and set water near the mixture. When the rodent tastes the flour, it will be convinced the powder is safe and will consume the cement. The water will harden the cement inside of the rodent. The rat may sample the powder one night to be sure it's safe and return for a full feast the next night. So give the powder time to work. Children and pets are unlikely to consume the cement because of the unpleasant taste, but always be careful to keep children and pets away from any poison.

A clean home, and a clean, orderly garage and attic will prevent all types of pests, including rodents. Food left on kitchen counters or in open food containers invites rodents and insects to invade your home. Once present, rodents can chew through cardboard containers, so if you have an infestation, store food in plastic or glass. Also check for holes in exterior walls that allow rodents or insects to enter.

Mosquitoes

The best defense against mosquitoes is good screens on windows and doors. Mosquito eggs require still water to develop — stagnant ponds, lakes, and salt marshes are effective breeding grounds. So is still water in rain gutters, an abandoned wagon or child's toy, a boat, or the dog's water dish. Eliminate all sources of standing water. Change water in the pet's bowl daily, and change water in a bird bath every three days. Wheelbarrows should be stored on end, and boats and tubs of water placed to avoid pooled water. Ponds or ornamental pools can be stocked with the Gambusia minnow, or mosquito fish, which eats mosquito larvae. Many cities will provide you with Gambusia minnows.

City-wide spraying of pesticides to prevent mosquitoes is a hazardous practice. But it's a cheap and easy solution to short-sighted city governments which fail to consider the larger picture. Mosquitoes can become resistant to neurotoxic pesticides, whereas birds, bats, and humans cannot. When birds and bats consume pesticide-infested insects, the poison gets concentrated as it moves up the food chain, because the bird or bat is exposed to the poison in each of the bugs it consumes. As a result, neurotoxic pesticides protect the mosquito by killing off nature's primary pest controllers.

As birds, bats, and the other natural insect predators are destroyed, people become increasingly dependent on toxic chemicals, which in turn become increasingly less effective as the mosquitoes develop resistance. When city mosquito abatement programs rely solely on neurotoxic pesticides, they are insuring future mosquito problems. Effective programs focus on source reduction, such as removing standing water and cleaning ditches; biological controls, such as bacterial larvicides; and natural preditors, such as the Gambusia minnow and dragon flies.

The best protection from mosquitoes is physical barriers, such as screens and protective clothing. A nontoxic repellent is citronella candles during an evening out of doors. Also, yellow outdoor light bulbs attract fewer bugs than white bulbs.

When you apply a neurotoxic bug repellent on your skin, some amount of the neurotoxin will enter your bloodstream. These products are capable of dissolving paint, varnish, and leather, so using them on human skin doesn't make a lot of sense.

If you read the directions of a neurotoxic repellent, it will tell you to apply only to exposed skin. A repellent should never be applied to skin covered by clothing, because of the risk of damage to the nervous system due to the clothing trapping it against the skin. Never apply these products to the hands of a child, because the child is likely to rub his mouth or eyes.

You can make your own non-neurotoxic mosquito repellents with citronella oil and pennyroyal oil, but their potency has to be diluted before applying to your skin. Dilute a few drops of these natural essential oils in an ounce of base. A nontoxic base of either vegetable oil or a grain alcohol like vodka (which is less toxic than rubbing alcohol) can be used.

Vinegar can also be applied to the skin as a repellent. Taking a daily dose of several hundred milligrams of vitamin B1 has been found to be effective by some people in preventing mosquito bites. And some have found that eating lots of garlic or rubbing garlic on the skin repels mosquitoes. Basil and tansy are garden plants that help repel mosquitoes.[28]

Flies

Flies are related to mosquitoes. Installing good screens and eliminating strong food odors will help keep them out of your home. Flies are attracted to garbage, so make sure the lids of your garbage cans fit snugly. Rotting fruit in the yard will also attract flies. Flies are repelled by oil of clove and citrus oil, so hanging out bunches of cloves or scratching the skin of an orange and leaving it out in the room can repel them. You can make nontoxic fly-paper by spreading a thin layer of honey on bright yellow paper. The color attracts the fly and the honey glues its feet to the paper.

Spiders are a fly's natural enemy, and their presence in your yard can help reduce this annoying pest. Most of all, don't forget the flyswatter![29]

Termites

Some of the most dangerous pesticides have been used in the war on termites. After New York State was confronted with the human health hazard and the environmental threat of chlordane — which can cause neurological and immunological effects more than twenty years after it is applied — they banned the use of this toxic, long-lasting pesticide. The state found that homes treated with highly toxic chlordane often needed to be retreated, and sometimes within one to two years of the initial treatment, for preventing or controlling infestations. Their recommendations included structural modifications, the use of termite-resistant wood, biological controls, and integrated pest management.[30]

If you're building a new home, here are some materials and methods to use. Termite-resistant woods include heart tidewater red cypress and heart redwood. Poured concrete is resistant to termites; a reinforced concrete cap four inches high between the foundation and the subflooring will expose termite tubes. Sand can be used as a barrier against termites if it is laid underneath the slab foundation. This method was incorporated into the building code in Honolulu in 1989. A heavy polyethylene sheet can also be placed under the concrete slab to act as a barrier, particularly in very moist regions. For an existing structure, sand can be applied to the outer surface of the foundation to protect against termite infestations originating outside the structure.

Make sure that wood debris is never mixed with the dirt used to fill underneath porches, steps, and patios. Wood scraps around the structure are believed to cause half of the infestations of subterranean termites. It's also important to have good water drainage so that water doesn't collect. Keeping the area underneath your home cold and dry will discourage a colony from developing. Unexcavated areas under the home need good cross-ventilation; eighteen-mesh metal screening can be used to cover openings under the house and in the attic. There can be adequate clearance between the structural wood and the soil, and there needs to be adequate room in the crawl space to inspect for termites.

The foundation walls and supporting piers should be constructed to minimize future cracks or fissures which termites could attack. To protect the structure, exterior wood should be at least six inches off the ground and wooden floor joists at least twenty-four inches off the ground.

In short, a building should be constructed to resist termites. Using a dangerous neurotoxin is a poor substitute for proper initial construction.

Doing an annual termite inspection will allow you to respond early to a termite problem. As with all pests, an early invasion is easier to combat than an established colony. If the infestation is limited to a small area, the infested wood can be cut out and replaced.

Termites can be baked out by heating an area up to 140 degrees for ten minutes with either a space heater or a heat lamp. Pest-killing heating equipment can be used to heat a home or building to 160 degrees. If your local pest control company doesn't know how to use heat to kill termites, call another company. Some companies also use electrical currents to kill termites.

If the infestation originates in a piece of furniture, remove the furniture from the property. You can then treat the infestation with heat or dispose of the item.[31]

Carpenter Ants

Carpenter ants tunnel into wood to nest. They can be successfully controlled with boric acid. Preventing moisture underneath the house will help impede an infestation.[32]

Conclusions

Effective pest control includes prevention, early detection, and appropriate action. The best prevention is a clean, well-maintained home that doesn't provide food, water, or shelter to unwanted pests. Leaky, moldy places in your house can attract many types of pests. Defective roofing, clogged rain gutters, leaky plumbing, and small cracks in walls all increase the risk of unwanted critters. Open garbage, unsealed foods, and cluttered places will also attract bugs.

By paying attention, you can detect a pest problem early. At the first sign of an invader, take action. Do not allow any type of infestation to build to a crisis level.

As you learn about the pests you're trying to get rid of, you'll learn how to send them packing. The goal is not to destroy the entire insect or rodent kingdom, just to keep them out of your home. Occasionally, appropriate action is to allow nature to take its course. In north Texas, for example, there's an annual invasion of crickets. Crickets cover the city, and they're so thick at night that you can't walk outside without stepping on them. In less than two weeks they're gone. If you poison your entire neighborhood, they leave. If you do nothing, they leave. They come for a short time and then they leave. Pesticides cannot stop the crickets, but they can harm the local birds, animals, and humans.

A WORD ABOUT EXTERMINATORS

Perhaps the most dangerous of all pest control techniques is to allow a nonlicensed exterminator—this includes you—to use neurotoxic pesticides in your home! While properly applied neurotoxins are a health threat, improperly applied neurotoxins can be deadly. It's easy to underestimate the toxic properties of neurotoxic pesticides, because they are available in every grocery and hardware store. Proper pest control requires knowledge of the pest and knowledge of the poison.

If you hire an exterminator, make sure that a qualified, licensed professional comes to your home, not an untrained assistant or unlicensed person who could disappear tomorrow. Use an exterminator who practices integrated pest management (IPM). IPM uses principles of prevention, early detection, and least toxic interventions prior to chemical interventions. An IPM exterminator should offer boric acid and natural pyrethrum treatments; boric acid is more effective against roaches than any neurotoxic pesticide. If the exterminator insists on using organophosphate, carbamate, chlorinated hydrocarbon pesticides, or synthetic pyrethrums in your home, look for a more qualified professional. An exterminator's insistence on using neurotoxins is a sign of poor knowledge about pest control resources. The EPA, some state and local governments, and Bio-Integral Resource Center (BIRC) will help train exterminators in IPM, so don't accept ignorance as an excuse.[33]

Before you let an exterminator use any substance in your home, ask about all of the chemicals that will be used, including inert ingredients (discussed on page 118). Get a written guarantee stating which chemicals will and will not be used.

Landlords would be well advised to make sure boric acid is used for pest control on their property, because neurotoxic pesticides have the potential to injure a tenant and lead to a liability lawsuit. Even if the landlord wins the lawsuit, the legal expenses and time spent make it a costly victory. It doesn't make sense to use high-risk techniques when safe, effective, low-cost alternatives are available.

As a tenant, it's important to know what form of pest control is being used in your home or business. You can request that boric acid and IPM techniques be used. Sometimes an owner will allow the renter to be responsible for pest control. If the owner requires the use of neurotoxic chemicals, think about whether you need to relocate, especially if anyone living or working in the building is experiencing health problems related to neurotoxicity. As an employer, you can be held liable for chemical injuries employees sustain on the job.

∽

We've covered only a brief summary of non-neurotoxic pest control. More information is available at bookstores, libraries, gardening societies, some gardening centers, in organic gardening journals, and on the Internet. You don't have to harm yourself or your family to eliminate pests if you know the nontoxic alternatives.

CHAPTER TWELVE

NONTOXIC PERSONAL PRODUCTS AND COSMETICS

onsider how intimate cosmetic products are. We rub soaps and lotions all over our skin. We use toothpastes, lip balms, and deodorants. Women apply make-up to their faces, eyes, and lips. Laundry products on our clothes have continual contact with our skin. Because chemicals on the surface of the skin can enter directly into the bloodstream, neurotoxic cosmetic products can pose a risk, even when they are highly diluted.

Most of us believe the ingredients in cosmetics are monitored for safety or regulated by the FDA. Here's the truth: Of the 3,410 cosmetic ingredients used in 1984, a complete health hazard assessment could be made on 2 percent of them. This means that reliable, scientific data about safety existed for 69 ingredients. No toxicity information at all was available for 1,909 ingredients used in cosmetic products! Some information was available for the other 1,432 ingredients.[1]

Although the FDA has jurisdiction over cosmetics, their authority is remarkably limited. According to the FDA *Cosmetics Handbook*:

> Approval by the FDA is not required to market a cosmetic in the United States. With the exception of color additives and

some prohibited or restricted ingredients, cosmetic manufacturers may, on their own responsibility, use essentially any raw material as a cosmetic ingredient and market the product without approval.[2]

This means that with few exceptions, manufacturers are free to use any ingredient they choose. Some of the neurotoxic ingredients used in cosmetics include solvents such as benzene and toluene, methyl ethyl ketone, acetone, ammonia, isopropyl alcohol, and preservatives such as formaldehyde, quaternium 15, imidazolidinyl urea, methylchloroisothiazolinone/methylisothiazolinone (MCI/MI), and thimerosal.[3]

There is one ingredient listed on most consumer products that appears innocuous, almost friendly, but it's the most deceptive of all—the ingredient called "fragrance" discussed in chapter 10. Fragrance can refer to any combination of thousands of chemicals. According to literature from the FDA, there are between 5,000 and 6,000 fragrance materials.[4] About 1,500 of these chemicals are commonly used. Manufacturers are not required to reveal the chemicals used in a fragrance (or a "flavor") to the FDA. A typical fragrance formula contains between 20 and 300 individual ingredients. Some formulas contain as many as 800 ingredients.[5] Most fragrance formulas contain neurotoxic ingredients, including acetone, phenolic compounds, alcohols, and numerous petroleum-based substances.

There are no accurate records of how many people are negatively affected by neurotoxic chemicals used in cosmetic products. One of the only symptoms monitored is skin irritation, or contact dermatitis. Fragrance is the primary ingredient in cosmetics that causes contact dermatitis, and the ingredient grouping "preservatives" is the second most frequent cause.[6]

Cases of contact dermatitis do not reveal neurotoxicity, however; they only reveal the product's potential to irritate the skin. If you're having a neurotoxic reaction to fragrances or other chemicals in your cosmetics, you could experience headaches, fatigue, forgetfulness, irritability, sleep problems, visual problems, or clumsiness. A child who is reacting to fragrances could be irritable, tired, forgetful, acting out, or unable to focus his thinking. These symptoms could persist throughout the day, not just when the product is used, because cosmetics remain on your skin all day. Some fragrances linger for days, even a week. If you reapply the product daily, you are never away from it, which means it could be difficult to link a symptom with a product. If you think you're experiencing neurotoxic symptoms, remove fragrance products from your routine for several days.

The most concentrated fragrance products are perfume, cologne, and aftershave. Many women find that their chronic headaches get "cured" when they quit wearing perfume. For a headache sufferer, it's certainly worth trying.

You don't have to stop wearing all cosmetics. Neither do you have to expose yourself to harmful toxic substances. Numerous product lines use natural, nontoxic ingredients in their cosmetic products. Many natural sources of fragrances are not harmful. Perfumes have been made for centuries, and it wasn't until this century that petroleum compounds (petrochemicals) were used in place of natural ingredients, making perfumes neurotoxic. It's the synthetic imitation of natural fragrances that's a threat to health.

If perfume is important to you, protect yourself by only using the real thing—fragrance from natural sources. Natural fragrances come from plant sources, such as real roses, lavender, mint, lemons, cinnamon, and others. These natural fragrances can be purchased in a concentrated form, known as a "natural essential oil." An "artificial essential oil" or a "perfume oil" is derived from petrochemicals.

A natural essential oil is quite concentrated. If you were to put it directly on your skin, it would burn. It has to be diluted in some type of base. You can select an oil base, such as almond oil or olive oil, or an alcohol base. Many commercial perfumes have a base of wood alcohol or acetone, which are neurotoxic. Instead, you can use a grain alcohol, like vodka, to dilute the essential oil. A couple drops of the natural essential oil in an ounce of base is all you need.[7]

Potpourri is made with either synthetic, petrochemical fragrance or with natural fragrance. If you enjoy potpourri, make sure the fragrance added to the dried petals and leaves is from natural plant sources. You may want to make your own potpourri, using a natural essential oil or a natural ingredient like real vanilla (see chapter 10 for other natural alternatives).

NONTOXIC COSMETICS

When selecting cosmetic products, look for products that have the ingredients you need without neurotoxic chemicals. "Fragrance" is an unnecessary, neurotoxic chemical. If a product is labeled "fragrance free," it will be less toxic than the scented counterpart. Products advertised as "natural" may contain fragrance, because "natural" is not an official designation, it's an advertising gimmick. Even products labeled "unscented" can have a fragrance to mask the scent of the actual product.

The following pages list companies that produce less toxic and nontoxic products. It's not a complete listing. The information is provided to help you find the kind of products you want and is not intended to endorse particular items.

Soap

We use soap on our skin every day. If there's a neurotoxic ingredient in your soap, it will enter your bloodstream.

Use real soap, which usually has a base of glycerin or of sodium hydroxide combined with animal fat or vegetable oil. Ingredients to avoid in soaps are fragrances and deodorants.

Plain soap and water are adequate to rinse away or kill most bacteria and eliminate body odor. Antibacterial soaps are an overkill product that expose you to unnecessary chemicals. The best defense against bacteria is to bathe and to wash your hands frequently. If you need a stronger bacteria killer (for example, if someone is sick), use hydrogen peroxide. It's deadly to germs without being dangerous to humans.

Nontoxic soaps available in the grocery store include Ivory soap and Neutrogena Unscented. Neutrogena is a glycerin soap that can quickly melt away. To prevent this in any glycerin soap, unwrap the bars when you bring them home from the store and leave them in the linen closet or somewhere else to dry out. The bars will appear to sweat but afterward will last about three times as long. There are numerous brands of pure soaps available in health food stores. A few of these are Simple Soap, Nature's Gate Vitamin E Soap, and fragrance-free Kiss My Face.

Lotions

Because lotions are lipid (fat) soluble, they can easily transport neurotoxins through your skin to your bloodstream. Your regular grocery store may carry a fragrance-free brand of lotion. At a health food store, there are several brands of lotions that are fragrance free or lightly scented with natural herbs. A natural moisturizer alternative is to use a vegetable or nut oil, such as almond oil. If you purchase almond oil in the cooking oil section of the store, you'll pay less for the same product purchased as a cosmetic. Health food stores also sell pure vitamin E oil, which can be used on your skin or lips. Vitamin E oil is a good substitute for petroleum jelly. You can also find vitamin E-based lip balms.

Makeup

Makeup comes in contact with highly sensitive areas of your skin, so it's important to find makeup that doesn't contain formaldehyde as a preservative, ammonia, or fragrance. Makeup labeled "hypoallergenic and fragrance free" is a reasonable alternative, because it doesn't contain fragrance or highly irritating chemicals. Two fragrance-free product lines sold in department stores are Almay and Unscented Clinique. The home distribution product line, Beauti-Control, carries some fragrance-free products, although their entire line is not fragrance free. In health food stores, fragrance-free and nontoxic makeup products are available from Paul Penders, Ida Grae, Aubrey Organics, and others.

Shampoo and Conditioner

Most larger health food stores sell a variety of brands of shampoo and conditioner without fragrance or other toxic ingredients. Here's a partial list: Granny's Rich and Radiant Shampoo and Conditioner (Granny's Old Fashioned Products), Simple Soap Shampoo, Kiss My Face Olive and Aloe Shampoo, and Tom's Natural Shampoo with Aloe & Almond (Tom's of Maine).

Hairspray

Hairspray can contain numerous neurotoxic chemicals. In department stores, less toxic options include fragrance-free or unscented hairsprays, which are available from Almay, Clinique, and AquaNet. In health food stores, natural hairsprays are available from Naturade, Aubrey Organics, VitaWave, and Earth Science. A nontoxic hairspray can be mail-ordered from the Living Source (see appendix A).

Deodorants

Many deodorants sold in the grocery store contain aluminum in addition to fragrance. Aluminum has been implicated as one cause of Alzheimer's disease. Since aluminum has no useful purpose in the body, it doesn't make sense to increase the amount of aluminum in your body by using this daily product on highly sensitive skin.

Most of the deodorants sold at health food stores do not contain aluminum, and they are scented with natural herbs rather than petrochemicals.

A couple brands are Nature's Gate and Tom's of Maine. Another alternative is Le Crystal Natural, which contains natural deodorant salts in a crystal form.

You can make your own deodorant by using baking soda or combining baking soda and corn starch. Corn starch also makes an excellent body powder in place of talcum powder.

Sunscreen

Sunscreen is another product that can contain neurotoxic chemicals, which pass through your skin into your bloodstream. Some brands of less toxic or nontoxic sunscreen sold in regular grocery stores or drugstores are: Safesun, Clinique, Ti, and Neutrogena. Nature's Gate, Aubrey Organics, and Mill Creek produce sunscreens, available through health food stores.

Shaving Cream

Men will want to find a shaving cream free of neurotoxic chemical additives. In regular grocery stores, some of your favorite brands may offer an unscented shaving cream. These brands probably contain a masking fragrance, but the amount of fragrance will be considerably less than the regular product. In health food stores, Aubrey Organics, Paul Penders, Tom's of Maine, and Kiss My Face all offer nontoxic shaving products.

Toothpaste

Health food stores carry several brands of toothpaste that don't contain benzyl alcohol, saccharin, colors, fluoride, and other harmful ingredients. Tom's of Maine and Nature's Gate are two such brands. Baking soda can also be used in place of toothpaste.

Laundry Detergents

Because you're continually in contact with your clothes, your sheets, and your towels, it's important to launder them with nontoxic soaps and detergents. If you suffer from rashes or unexplained itching, the problem may clear up once you switch to nontoxic soap products. If your child has health problems or unexplained behavior problems, monitor his or her progress after switching to fragrance-free or natural laundry products.

In regular grocery stores, several name brand companies carry an unscented version of their detergent. Some "unscented" brands still contain significant amounts of fragrance, so let your nose guide you to the product with the least amount of fragrance. Sometimes a less expensive, generic store brand of detergent is unscented. One of the least toxic alternatives in regular grocery stores is Arm & Hammer Unscented Washing Soda. Arm & Hammer also produces a perfume- and dye-free detergent.

Several home distributor product lines have built a reputation around a high quality laundry soap. Some of these companies have added fragrance in recent years, although the companies claim the fragrance is from a natural source. The Neo-Life home distribution network continues to sell fragrance-free Green Soap and Rugged Red.

In health food stores, several companies sell laundry soaps without fragrances or other synthetic chemicals. Some of these product lines include Granny's Old Fashioned Products, Allen's Naturally, and Ecover. These same companies sell dishwashing liquids.

Twenty Mule Team Borax is a natural laundry booster and can be added to the wash cycle to brighten and freshen clothes.

Fabric Softeners

Manufacturers try to convince us to buy fabric softeners. These dryer sheets, liquids, and sprays are designed to reduce static cling in synthetics such as polyester, acrylic, and acetate, which are made from petrochemical sources. Fabric softeners treat the fabric with a chemical residue, which then has continual contact with your skin.

Does your fabric softener actually improve the quality of your life, or did you buy it because of a good advertising campaign? You may want to evaluate whether you need this product at all. By running several loads of laundry without the fabric softener, you can determine if it makes any difference. One comedian commented that he threw a facial tissue in the dryer because it cost less and did about as much good.

One of the primary causes of static cling is drying clothes for too long. If you have a lot of static cling, try running the dryer for a shorter period of time. It will save money on your utility bill as well as on fabric softener. Consider buying clothes made of natural fibers such as cotton, wool, and silk, which are not as prone to static cling. Wearing clothes made of natural rather than synthetic fibers will eliminate another exposure to petrochemicals. The least neurotoxic synthetic fibers are nylon and rayon.

If fabric softener is important to you, one alternative is to buy unscented dryer sheets, which are less toxic than scented dryer sheets or sprays. Nontoxic dryer sheets are available at health food stores from Ecover and Allen's Naturally.

Dry Cleaning

Dry-cleaning fluids contain solvents that are highly neurotoxic, such as 1,1,1-trichloroethane and trichloroethylene. Emissions from dry-cleaned clothes have been measured in homes, and they have been shown to be a significant source of indoor air pollution.[8]

Avoid dry cleaning as much as possible. When clothes have to be dry-cleaned, take precautions to protect the air in your home by not trapping solvent fumes inside. When you bring the dry-cleaned item home, remove the plastic bag before you even bring the garment into the house, and throw the bag in an outside garbage can. If possible, hang the item in a garage or outside porch to allow the solvents to evaporate before bringing the clothing into your home. It may take several days to a week. If you have to hang the garment inside, provide as much ventilation as possible.

While expensive suits and sequined evening gowns do need professional cleaning, many items labeled "dry clean only" can be laundered safely at home, particularly if they are hung to dry instead of being put in the dryer. As you purchase new clothes, you may want to select garments that don't require dry cleaning.

Paper Products
Another place to avoid fragrance, color, and added lotion is in toilet paper, facial tissues, and napkins. When these products come into contact with sensitive skin, added fragrances and colors could cause irritation.

Products for Children and Babies
It's never in the interest of an infant or child to be exposed to products with fragrance or other neurotoxins. To protect your infant from neurotoxins, be sure to use natural lotions, unscented or fragrance-free baby wipes, pure soaps, and other fragrance-free products. Corn starch is a natural powder that can be used in place of talcum powder. Vitamin E oil can be used in place of petroleum jelly.

Cotton diapers are the best choice from the standpoint of neurotoxicity, waste disposal, diaper rash, and cost. You can soak diapers in a mixture of warm water and a half cup of borax to reduce odor and staining. To kill bacteria, wash diapers in hot water and dry for forty minutes on the hottest setting. If you have a clothesline, sunlight also acts as a natural disinfectant.[9] Some people prefer to use a diaper service. You can find services that do not use strong chemical detergents or add fragrances. Some services provide a choice of more than one cleaning process.

If you're using disposable diapers, be sure to use an unscented brand. Sometimes a store's generic brand diaper is unscented, whereas name-brand diapers can have strong chemical fragrances. The chemicals in certain brands of disposable diapers expose the developing brain of a baby to unnecessary neurotoxins.

∽

Because products used on your skin enter your bloodstream, only items safe enough to be used *in* your body should be used *on* your body. Use nontoxic products on you skin to reduce the amount of neurotoxins your body has to detoxify. You can find fragrance-free and nontoxic products with some effort, but it will be well worth the investment. You may notice an improvement in your health or the health of your child as you eliminate this potential source of neurotoxins.

CHAPTER THIRTEEN

TOXIN-FREE FOOD

Many people think they should eat healthier food, but they're afraid it means eating alfalfa sprouts, tofu, rice cakes, and granola. The truth is, you can significantly improve your diet by reducing the chemicals in your food.

MAKING SMART CHOICES

Food grown without neurotoxic chemicals is labeled *certified organic*. Sometimes people confuse the designation of *organic* with words like *natural* or *health food,* or they associate it with low-fat or vegetarian foods. What do all these labels mean?

Organic Food

Organic food is grown without neurotoxic pesticides or synthetic fertilizers. If an apple is grown on a tree treated with some type of pesticide, it has been grown commercially, not organically. Unless it is specially designated as certified organic, the produce in grocery stores is commercially grown.

With commercially grown food, many chemical treatments are applied to the seed or to the soil rather than to the exterior of the plant.

Fertilizers, herbicides, insecticides, and fungicides will move from the soil into the plant. These toxins are incorporated into the cells of the plant, just as they're incorporated into the cells of your body. You can wash off chemical residues on the surface which may be applied during shipping and storage, but you can't eliminate a pesticide residue inside the fruit. There is no form of preparation that can make a commercially grown apple organic.

If that same apple had been grown on a tree not treated with neurotoxic pesticides, and if no pesticides had been used in recent years, then it would be organic. For a meat to be organic, the animal has to be fed organic feed and not given shots of hormones or antibiotics.

Organic food is real food. It hasn't been contaminated with neurotoxic pesticides, treated with other types of chemicals, or injected with hormones or antibiotics. Organic food is what we were designed to consume, and all of us need to make our diets as organic as possible.

If you've eaten organic food, you've probably noticed how good it tastes. Organic produce tends to be more flavorful than commercial food, perhaps because it was allowed to vine ripen, or perhaps because real food that isn't treated with chemicals is just better! Sometimes organic food isn't as pretty or perfect looking as commercial food. But it's real, and this is apparent in the taste.

Health Food
Healthy and *health food* are wholesome sounding terms that mean anything and nothing on a product label. The term *health food* may simply mean food that is bought at the health food store. People often associate granola, yogurt-covered almonds, and alfalfa sprouts with health food. In fact, health foods may or may not be healthy, and they may or may not be organic. Health food stores, however, are an important resource because they usually sell some organic foods and natural cosmetic products. Health food is an industry, and a wise consumer must evaluate the products of this industry.

Natural
The word *natural* on a label can mean almost anything. Many times it's a labeling gimmick. Sometimes companies deceptively use the

term *natural flavoring* in their list of ingredients to hide the fact that they're using MSG. Many times *natural* is used to indicate that a food product contains real food ingredients and doesn't contain chemical additives. Other times it refers to food that actually is organic but hasn't been certified. To be certified, a farmer has to pay the state to certify that his land is organic. Local organic gardeners are unlikely to be certified.

The only time *natural* is an actual designation is in regard to meat. Many health food stores label meat as *natural* when the animal was fed grass or regular commercial feed but wasn't given injections of hormones or antibiotics. Natural meat is a healthier choice than commercial meat. The extensive use of hormones and antibiotics in meats and milk products has led to increasing concerns about its impact on humans. About 9.9 million pounds of antibiotics were used in animal production in 1985. Food animals are currently the largest single source of antibiotic resistant salmonellae.[1]

Low-Fat
Low-fat food is the current fad in food sales. *Low-fat* and *nonfat* labels abound, but what they mean varies from product to product. Some foods that have never contained fat—beans, pastas, and grains—are labeled *nonfat* as a selling point. Although some low-fat and nonfat products are healthy, many foods are labeled nonfat because chemicals have been substituted for real food. Some companies have made responsible substitutions to reduce fat, such as using yogurt in place of sour cream.

Our bodies are designed to convert a reasonable amount of fat into useful fatty acids, but there's no biological benefit to ingesting synthetic chemicals. Unlike essential fatty acids, which are used in building cells and storing energy, chemical additives can only deplete cell resources as the body tries to detoxify from them. Although our bodies are able to detoxify some quantity of these synthesized compounds, they have no use in our bodies.

Vegetarian
A vegetarian diet does not include meats. Some vegetarians eliminate all animal products, including eggs and dairy. Some people are

vegetarians for health reasons, some have convictions about the amount of land required to raise beef as opposed to grains, and some people are vegetarian due to religious convictions. A vegetarian diet may or may not be organic.

Allergy Diets

An allergy diet eliminates certain foods or food additives that cause a person to have specific symptoms. Some food allergies can resolve with time, which means that if a person avoids a certain food, it may be added back into the diet later without problems. When children have health problems, a doctor or nutritionist may have parents withhold certain foods or food additives to see if the foods contribute to the problem. Food additives, such as a food coloring, can cause striking behavioral responses in certain children.[2] Sometimes foods are withheld for other reasons. For example, if a young child has frequent ear infections, milk products may be withheld to reduce a mucus buildup which could breed future infections.

CHEMICALS IN OUR FOOD

People mistakenly believe that the EPA or FDA is carefully monitoring our food to make sure harmful chemicals do not affect us. This is not the case.

Pesticides

There are 20,000 pesticide products registered under the Federal Pesticide Law. The EPA estimates that an average of 3.2 pounds of pesticides per person are used in agriculture each year.[3] The National Research Council panel concluded in 1984 that a complete health hazard assessment could be conducted on only 10 percent of the 3,350 ingredients in pesticide production![4] This estimate was based on information which was publicly available at the time. By 1987, 30 percent of insecticides, 50 percent of herbicides, and 90 percent of fungicides were found to cause tumors in laboratory animals.[5]

As alarming as these statistics are, they still underestimate the actual human health hazard. Scientific tests and legislative regulations continue to consider each pesticide individually.[6] When produce sold in grocery stores is tested for pesticide residues, often more than one pesticide residue is found. These studies do not consider the synergistic effects of a combination of neurotoxins, nor do they consider the accumulation of the chemicals in our bodies. The scientific studies conducted measure rates of cancer, but they do not measure for neurotoxicity. These pesticides are specifically developed for their neurotoxic properties, yet there's no testing for behavioral problems, learning problems, and the slow degeneration of brain cells.[7]

Of the over 3,000 chemicals in pesticide formulations that can be used on foods, which should be tested first? Which poses the greatest danger? In 1989 there was a public outcry over Alar, a chemical used to make apples ripen. At the same time, dialifos was being used to control insects and mites in apples, citrus, grapes, nuts, potatoes, and vegetables. Dialifos is chemically related to thalidomide, the drug that caused children to be born with deformed arms and legs. The potential of dialifos to cause birth defects and its teratology was unknown.[8] Were these two neurotoxins more dangerous than the other 3,348?

It appears that neurotoxic chemicals are assumed innocent until proven guilty beyond a reasonable doubt. Once approved, these chemicals will not be removed from the marketplace unless there is enormous public opposition. The EPA did not take action against Alar until the public outcry in 1989, even though they had evidence that it posed a cancer risk to children in the 1970s.[9] DDT continues to be produced and sent to foreign countries, even though it's banned in this country.

Neurotoxic chemicals used in food production contribute to the accumulation of neurotoxins within all of us. Some people are able to detoxify from neurotoxins efficiently, but some experience chronic health problems such as fatigue, immuno-suppression, or endocrine disorders. Some experience silent brain damage until the loss is so extensive that it shows itself in the form of neurodegenerative disease. And some experience damage to their DNA, which leads to cancer or birth defects in their children. Neurotoxins in food sources carry a high price tag.

Excitotoxins

Clear and convincing scientific and medical data is not adequate to protect the public from highly profitable food additives. These chemicals continue to be used in foods, despite public objection.

Food additives known as excitotoxins are amino acids (the building blocks of protein) which can excite sensitive nerve cells to the point of death.[10] These additives may be the most blatant example of how the value of human health has been superseded by the goal of financial gain. The dangerous excitotoxic food additives include monosodium glutamate (MSG), aspartame (NutraSweet), L-cysteine, and hydrolyzed vegetable protein (created through a process that releases both glutamate and aspartate from proteins).

MSG is the sodium salt of glutamic acid, an amino acid. Aspartame is a combination of two amino acids, phenylalanine and aspartate. Here's the problem. When amino acids occur naturally in foods, they are combined with other amino acids that allow them to be properly digested and used by the body. A protein, for example, could be a complex combination of as many as a thousand amino acids. The excitotoxic food additives flood the body with single amino acids, a situation the body is not designed to handle.

How do MSG and Aspartame affect brain functioning? Your brain uses both glutamate and aspartate as neurotransmitters (to communicate between cells). MSG consumption could cause too much glutamate to accumulate in your brain. As you may remember from chapter 3, the accumulation of too much of a neurotransmitter can have devastating consequences. Too much of the neurotransmitter acetylcholine is the cause of death from chemical warfare. Too much of the neurotransmitter dopamine is believed to cause schizophrenia.

MSG has the potential to change the balance of glutamate in the brain. There is increasing scientific evidence that excess glutamate can slowly kill the nerve cells that depend on it for communication. This slow, degenerative damage appears to be linked to Alzheimer's disease, Parkinson's disease, and ALS. For a more thorough and technical explanation of the impact of glutamate, read *Excitotoxins: The Taste that Kills* by the neurosurgeon Russell Blaylock, M.D.

Aspartate also acts as an excitatory neurotransmitter in the brain, so its potential to harm nerve cells is similar to glutamate. NutraSweet is composed of 40 percent aspartate and about 50 percent phenylalanine. Some people do not have the enzyme needed to metabolize phenylalanine. There is an inherited condition known as phenylketonuria (PKU), which hospitals test for at birth. If an infant or child with PKU eats foods with high levels of phenylalanine, the phenylalanine will accumulate to a toxic level and cause permanent brain damage such as mental retardation and seizures. Due to the risk of immediate, severe brain damage to people with PKU, the presence of NutraSweet is generally indicated on packages. But it can be served in restaurant food without warning. Unless you're tested, you wouldn't know if you're a PKU carrier, which could mean that you have a lowered capacity to metabolize phenylalanine.

Naturally occurring phenylalanine is an important substance because it's a precursor to the neurotransmitters dopamine and norepinephrine.[11] Too much phenylalanine, however, can lower the threshold for seizures.[12] This is of particular concern to pilots because it can make them susceptible to "flicker vertigo," which means that flashing lights (such as on runways and instrument panels) can trigger seizures.[13]

The third ingredient in NutraSweet (about 10 percent) is methyl alcohol. Methyl alcohol, or wood alcohol, is a household disinfectant you were probably told not to drink because it could cause blindness. Hundreds of people have complained of experiencing visual problems as a result of consuming NutraSweet.[14]

The Searle company faced many difficulties from 1969 to 1981 in getting aspartame approved. Early studies of aspartame demonstrated a high incidence of brain tumors in test animals.[15] This problem allegedly was solved in later studies by removing tumors from live animals, presenting false values, and substituting healthy animals for sick ones.[16]

In another early study of aspartame on monkeys, all of the animals exposed to medium or high doses of NutraSweet experienced grand mal seizures.[17] This finding was not investigated further. Early findings of uterine polyps, ovarian tumors, and altered blood cholesterol were reportedly withheld from the FDA.[18] Studies of bladder cancer (primarily a concern for males) were only performed on female mice.[19]

Despite the unanimous 1980 decision by the Public Board of Inquiry to recommend banning aspartame for human consumption, it was approved in 1981 as a "food additive." This designation means that it's exempt from all future safety monitoring. In 1983, it was approved for use in soft drinks. Between 1973 and 1990, the incidence of brain tumors increased 67 percent in people over 65 and 10 percent in all age groups. The greatest increases occurred in 1985–1987.[20]

The symptoms that have been associated with NutraSweet consumption include: headache, seizures, confusion and memory loss, visual problems, and blindness.[21] The neurotoxicity of NutraSweet increases when it is in liquid form or when it is heated.[22] For a more thorough review of NutraSweet read *Aspartame (NutraSweet®), Is It Safe?* by internist H. J. Roberts, M.D.

Under no circumstances should infants or children be given foods containing NutraSweet or MSG. Pregnant women will want to protect their babies from these excitotoxins—which appear able to pass through the placenta and through breast milk—by avoiding them. Giving a child food containing MSG or NutraSweet would be like giving him a low-dose psychiatric drug that changes the biochemistry of his brain. A child's developing brain cannot withstand the chemical assaults an adult might be able to deflect.

One study of the impact of MSG on the developing brain found that rats exposed to MSG for eleven days after birth were shorter, fatter, exhibited hyperactive behavior, and had difficulty escaping from mazes.[23] There is no FDA ban on using MSG in baby food, so examine the ingredients to be sure MSG is not hidden under a disguised name (see below).

As with all neurotoxic chemicals, there are individual differences among people in their ability to detoxify. The young, the elderly, and people who are sick will be especially vulnerable to excitotoxins. NutraSweet can also pose a significant risk by interacting with other drugs.[24]

You may wonder why food manufacturers would want to use these dangerous products. It's simple: Artificial sweeteners are highly lucrative, and NutraSweet has revitalized the diet soft drink industry. MSG also serves an important function. It is able to disguise low-grade, poor quality foods. It works by changing your perception of how food tastes.

MSG can legally be listed under multiple names on food labels, so you may not know when it's been added to processed foods. This practice is a deliberate deception by food manufacturers. The willingness of the FDA to allow this practice is disturbing because it violates your right to know what you're buying. The following table lists the aliases of MSG.

ADDITIVES THAT ALWAYS CONTAIN MSG [25]	ADDITIVES THAT FREQUENTLY CONTAIN MSG	ADDITIVES THAT MAY CONTAIN MSG
Monosodium glutamate	Flavoring	Soy protein concentrate
Sodium caseinate	Bouillon	Enzymes
Hydrolyzed vegetable protein	Natural flavoring	Soy protein isolate
	Broth	Carrageenan
Calcium caseinate	Natural beef or chicken flavoring	Whey protein concentrate
Hydrolyzed protein		
Plant protein extract	Stock	
Hydrolyzed plant protein	Malt flavoring	
Textured protein	Spices	
Hydrolyzed oat flour	Malt extract	
Yeast extract	Seasoning	
Autolyzed yeast		

Other Food Additives

The National Research Council panel estimated in 1984 that a complete health hazard assessment could be conducted on only 5 percent of 8,627 food additives.[26] Synthetic food colors are added to foods to make them appear more appealing, particularly in breakfast cereals and other foods created to appeal to children. FD&C colors are made from coal tar.[27] There is scientific evidence that some children react to synthetic food coloring with hyperactivity, irritability, restlessness, and sleep disturbances. Tartrazine (a food color) has also been implicated in precipitating asthma, eczema, hives and swelling, and migraine.[28]

Artificial flavors are another source of added chemicals and potential neurotoxins in our food. There are more than 1,500 petrochemical-derivative flavoring agents,[29] and the FDA does not require companies to reveal the ingredients in "flavors" (or in "fragrances"). This means that ingredients such as "imitation strawberry" or "lemon flavoring" are basically unregulated by the FDA. Artificial flavorings are used by food manufacturers because they're cheaper than the real thing—imitation vanilla costs less than real vanilla.

Another source of food additives are preservatives such as BHT, BHA, TBHQ, sodium benzoate, nitrites and nitrates. Some scientific studies have demonstrated substantial improvement in some children with hyperactivity and attention deficit disorder when artificial colors, flavors, and preservatives were eliminated from their diets.[30] Food additives are recognized as a widespread source of neurotoxins for both children and adults.[31]

You can reduce your exposure to neurotoxic chemicals in foods by selecting items that only contain real food ingredients.

HOW TO GET STARTED

Eating 100 percent organic food would benefit all of us. We were designed to eat the real thing, not chemical substitutions. The place to start learning about organic foods is usually at a health food store. Some stores carry only vitamins and supplements, so look for one that is actually a grocery store. If you live in a large city, there may be a large health food store that is comparable to a regular grocery store. Most towns have small stores, which can be expensive. If you live in a rural community, there may be an organic farm where you can purchase organic produce. In some parts of the country you can purchase organic dairy products and produce from Mennonite and Amish farmers, who do not use pesticides.

Remember that just because a store claims to sell health food doesn't mean that every product on the shelf is healthy. An expensive, gourmet food that is not organic may contain as many chemical additives as the cheap discount version at a regular grocery store. Look for organic food, not overpriced food.

With processed foods, the box can be labeled *organic* if only one ingredient is organic, while harmful additives like MSG can still be in the product. If the primary ingredients or the majority of the ingredients are not organic, then the labeling is deceptive. The word *organic* should appear before each individual ingredient that is organic, unless the product is labeled *100 percent organic ingredients*.

If you start looking at organic foods sold in a health food store, you can become familiar with brand names and companies that carry these products. Most people are not able to eat a 100 percent organic diet, but even having part of your diet organic is a benefit. You may find that your health improves as you eat more foods that are free from contaminants.

For most people, the cost of organic food is the biggest constraint. You can begin by buying organic items competitively priced with commercial food. Some stores will let you order a case (usually twelve items) for a discount. You can also save money buying organic food through a co-op. By bargain hunting, you can find ways to increase the amount of organic food in your diet while staying within your budget.

Produce

Large grocery store chains are now carrying a few organic produce items. But most organic produce is sold in health food stores, at a farmers' market, or directly from an organic farm. At a farmers' market, you can ask the grower how they keep bugs off their produce. Most Mennonite and Amish farmers do not use pesticides, so their produce could be organic, even if it's not certified.

Different environmental and consumer groups measure the level of pesticides found in different foods. Learning which foods are the most contaminated could help you know how to prioritize your shopping. You may want to grow your own organic produce.

Dry Goods

Organic bulk items such as rice, flour, pastas, and legumes are often competitively priced in health food stores. Having these important staples be organic can improve your health and the health of your family.

Often you find the best price on these items through an organic food co-op. Some co-ops are food stores where members receive discounts on groceries. Other co-ops deliver orders for several families at a pick-up site where members divide the orders. Buying in bulk gets you a better price. Look in your phone book or ask health-conscious friends to help you locate these small co-ops. Major co-op distribution companies for different regions in the country are listed in appendix B. The regional distributor should be able to help you find a local co-op.

Meat and Dairy

The best meat is organic meat from animals that were fed organic feed and were not given hormones or antibiotics. This meat can be purchased from an organic farmer and at some health food stores. Many health food stores also sell "natural meat," which comes from animals that may have eaten commercial feed but were not given hormones or antibiotics. Coleman beef is a well-recognized brand of natural and organic beef.

In some parts of the country, natural chicken can be purchased at a regular grocery store from producers who do not use hormones or antibiotics. Usually these producers will advertise the natural way they raise their chickens. Many health food stores sell natural or organic poultry. Sometimes you can buy organic eggs from someone who raises chickens organically in their back yard.

Organic dairy products are available in many health food stores. Since most Mennonite and Amish farmers do not use pesticides, their dairy products are often organic. It's worth the effort to locate organic milk and butter because cows, like all mammals, concentrate neurotoxins in their milk.

Packaged Foods

More and more processed organic foods are available in wholesale operations. If you buy at a health food store, you can reduce the cost of packaged organic foods by buying in bulk. Many stores will allow you to order a case at a reduced price. The best way to obtain packaged organic foods at a reasonable price may be to join an organic food co-op (see appendix B).

Organic baby food is available at health food stores and through food co-ops. Feeding your baby organic food will give your child a healthy head start.

Condiments

Spices should be purchased at a health food store and checked to be sure they haven't been irradiated. You can purchase canning salt or sea salt, which doesn't have chemical ingredients to prevent caking. If you add a couple grains of organic rice to your salt shaker to absorb the moisture, your salt will not cake.

Natural, cold-pressed oils are a healthy alternative to lard or non-stick chemical sprays. Salad dressings, sauces, soups, gravy mixes, and frozen diet foods are often particularly high in MSG, so these would be good items to purchase at a health food store. Check the label, however, because some health food companies disguise MSG with other names.

For sweeteners, use real foods such as honey, fruit, and sugar, rather than NutraSweet or saccharine.

Storage and Cookware

As you work on locating chemical-free food, you'll want to store and cook foods in materials that do not emit neurotoxins. The best material for storing food is glass. Plastics, particularly soft plastics, can emit hydrocarbons. If you do use plastic, wet foods, such as juices, will absorb more of the plastic residue than hard dried foods, such as rice. Many natural and organic canned foods come in cans lined with enamel to prevent the tin or lead soldering from leaching into the food. Aluminum and Teflon cookware can emit neurotoxins, whereas cookware made of glass, glass/ceramic, and stainless steel will not.

DIETING AND WEIGHT CONTROL

Some diet programs include prepackaged foods that contain many chemical ingredients. When you eat these kinds of artificial foods, you're increasing the detoxification demands on your body while depriving it of nutritional resources. You would never expect your car to run on water in place of fuel. Likewise, it's not reasonable to demand that your body function without real nutrition.

Reasonable weight-loss programs recommend increased exercise and a healthy, balanced diet. Weight-loss programs that actually work usually recommend three meals a day plus two or three snacks.

Skipping meals is an unhealthy practice that can make it harder to lose weight. Consistently supplying your body with the nutrients it needs will reduce craving and bingeing.

Many people need to take better care of their bodies by eating regularly and eating foods that are good for them, not punishing themselves or depriving their bodies of needed nutrients. Rapid weight loss is not healthy. Among other health concerns, the fat cells often store neurotoxins, and releasing too many of them at once could cause neurotoxic symptoms.

Do not be deceived that NutraSweet will help you lose weight. The sweet taste will stimulate your body to release insulin and other neurotransmitters. When the expected calories do not arrive, your brain will signal increased hunger, and your natural response to this urgent need is to eat and drink more sugar and simple carbohydrates. The American Cancer Society documented that people who use artificial sweeteners gain more weight than those who avoid them.[32]

At the time of writing this book, a newscast announced that the FDA had approved a new food additive. This one is an imitation fat called Olestra. In a television news interview about this new product, a scientist explained how Olestra robs the body of important nutrients. The public-relations spokesperson for the company glibly replied this wasn't important. She explained how they could add extra nutrients to food, and she went as far as to say that losing beta-carotene was not important, because we don't know what its purpose is in the body.

Do not be deceived by a company that wants your money and has no regard for your health. We need the naturally occurring nutrients in real food, whether or not scientists have figured out how our bodies use them. A successful weight loss plan has to work *with* your body, not against it.

ENJOYING FOOD

Advice about diets and nutrition abound! Rather than offer specific nutritional advice, I recommend that you reduce your exposure to neurotoxins by eating organic foods as much as possible.

Sometimes people think they'll have to eat unfamiliar or

unpleasant foods if they eat organically. An organic diet can include hamburgers, spaghetti, and many other familiar foods you're comfortable with. Organic frozen pizza, organic chocolate chip cookies, and organic potato chips are all available. An organic diet can include high-fiber foods or high-fat foods, but it will not include neurotoxins.

A sudden, radical change in the way you and your family eat may cause stress and frustration. Sometimes husbands and kids resent it when mom no longer allows them to eat the foods they're used to. Unless there's a medical concern that requires immediate attention, a gradual transition is usually more successful.

∽

Eating healthy foods should be enjoyable, not feel like a punishment. If you're being advised about diet changes by someone who is negative about foods and isn't providing you with positive choices, look for someone who can help you make reasonable, positive choices. Food is good, and we should be able to enjoy the real thing.

CHAPTER FOURTEEN

CHOICES IN MEDICINE

For most of us, our first memories of being ill include the loving nurture of our caregivers. We may remember the gentle hand and the cool cloth on our feverish foreheads. We can't assume we'll find the same thing in professional health care. Medicine is big business.

Professionals make their living by selling their skills or their products. Independent health practitioners are professional small business owners. Many are hired by large organizations to provide specified services. Professionals who are hired by a company or an insurance agency, have a loyalty to their employer, and this loyalty may or may not be in your best interest.

When you're a patient, you're the consumer who has to choose your health care. Many people choose to cooperate passively. But whatever choice a person makes, it's the person, not the health-care provider, who will live with the consequences.

TRADITIONAL MEDICINE

Traditional, conservative training programs for medical doctors focus on prescribing drugs and performing surgery. Their training generally does not include nutrition, prevention, herbal medicine, or neurotoxicity. If you break a bone, need a prescription medication, or need surgery, an MD is well qualified to help you. If you need to find out if you have a deficiency in vitamins or minerals, if your diet is contributing to health problems, if neurotoxic chemicals are contributing to health problems, or how to use natural preventive medicines, you may need to consult someone who has appropriate training in these fields.

Unfortunately, when it comes to preventive medicine, medical doctors are not in a good position to judge which preventive measures are successful. Think about it: Healthy people do not make appointments to see them. The role of a doctor is to intervene when prevention has been unsuccessful.

When consulting with a doctor, it's reasonable to get information about the health problem: What causes it? How can it be prevented? What are the treatment options? What is the prescribed treatment? A good doctor will want you to be well-informed, because only then can you follow the treatment program.

It's important to ask questions of your health-care professional. Many people find they don't have enough face-to-face time with their doctors to get their questions answered. When you consult with your doctor, present facts clearly and concisely. If you come with a checklist, most doctors will allow you to finish the list as long as you are brief and to the point. You may want to bring a concise, written medical history so a rushed doctor can scan previous health conditions and treatments.

Medications
There are numerous medical books, written for lay people, to inform you about your medical diagnosis and any medications prescribed for you. Or you can read the same medical textbooks or articles your doctor reads. Your local library will probably be a good source of medical information. If you live near a medical school, the library there will have excellent resources. You can find the majority of research on neurotoxic chemicals in the literature for industrial or occupational medicine, neuropsychology, behavioral toxicology, and environmental medicine. The more informed you are about your condition, the better equipped you will be at making the medical choices that are right for you.

The use of any medication, whether it is prescribed or over-the-counter, needs to be evaluated. As one doctor observed, "The trouble is that an agent that has powerful biological effects . . . has powerful biological effects."[1] There is always a cost/benefit ratio, and you want to be sure that the benefit is greater than the cost. It's not healthy to take excessive amounts of any medicine, prescription or over-the-counter. Be sure you actually need a medication before you take it. When you receive a prescription, check to see that the drug you get at the pharmacy is the right dosage of the drug you were prescribed. Read the printout provided with the prescription. If you have questions, ask the pharmacist. Many pharmacists will answer questions over the phone.

In selecting over-the-counter medications, consider the dyes, flavorings, and added ingredients. For example, NutraSweet is added to some laxatives. You would do better to make dietary changes, eat dried fruits, or take a natural laxative like psyllium (without added chemicals) than to rely on a drug. If you're dependent on over-the-counter medications or painkillers, maybe you need to find the cause, not just cover the symptoms.

When you cover up symptoms with medications in place of finding an underlying cause, you cover up an important signal of disease or injury. Sometimes a person's lifestyle causes their health problems. If someone is being exposed to neurotoxic chemicals at work, for example, taking aspirin for headaches may temporarily remove the pain while the injury continues. If this headache gets worse, and a doctor prescribes a stronger painkiller, the chemical injury continues to progress. Reducing chemical exposures at work and increasing detoxification, not painkillers, is what's needed. The only way to cure the problem is to find its source.

Emotional Support

A doctor who is unwilling to listen to your concerns or take your complaints seriously is probably not going to be able to help you. Remember, you're the consumer. You deserve to be treated with dignity and respect. If your doctor disrespects you or attacks your credibility, see someone else.

Sometimes people expect their doctors to provide them emotional support. Do not come to your doctor expecting a long, soothing conversation or consolation. A psychologist, counselor, social worker, or minister is better suited and trained to provide emotional support. Chronic pain is a tremendous source of stress. If you have chronic health problems, finding good emotional and social support to help you grieve your losses and learn better stress management skills is an important component in your ability to cope and recover.

Professionals in different specialties receive different types of training. No one is competent in all of the healing arts. It's not even a reasonable expectation. It is reasonable to expect professionals to recognize their own limitations and to refer you to other specialists when appropriate. This, however, does not always happen, so you'll want to be an active participant in decisions regarding your health and the health of your family.

ALTERNATIVE MEDICINE

An increasing number of people are turning to natural forms of medicine, with a focus on prevention, strengthening the immune system, diet, nutrition, vitamins and minerals, and the use of herbs and enzymes. Many people have benefited from using these natural techniques. Natural medicine, however, is also a for-profit business, so consumers need to be informed in this arena as well.

Some people view natural medicine as unconventional or ineffective. One stereotype commonly believed is that the use of herbs and other supplements involves incense and Eastern mysticism. A second stereotype is that most of these products are modern-day snake oil that just don't work.

Herbal Medicine
Through the centuries, people of every culture and religion have used herbs. Herbal medicine was the standard from which we departed with the discovery of penicillin. Now synthetic drugs have replaced medicinal herbs to a large extent in Western culture. But there is a return to these time-proven remedies as synthetic drugs have proven less effective in curing what ails us. Many of the "new" discoveries in natural medicine have been used for centuries. Midwives, for

example, are certainly not new, but increasingly they are in demand as women refuse to accept a medical model that deals with childbirth as if it were a disease.

An ancient healing herb used by Native Americans was white willow bark. The Reverend Edward Stone tried this medicinal bark in the 1700s. At that time, there was a philosophy in European medicine called the "doctrine of signatures." This philosophy held that nature provided cures for the sicknesses of the area. Reverend Stone reported to the Royal Society of England in 1763:

> As this tree delights in a moist or wet soil, where agues (chills and fevers) chiefly abound, the general maxim that many natural maladies carry their cures along with them or that their remedies lie not far from the causes . . . that this might be the intention of Providence here, I must own, had some little weight with me.[2]

In the 1850s, a chemist named Charles von Gerhardt created a synthesized version of white willow bark. Another chemist, Felix Hoffman, found this compound in the 1890s and gave it to his arthritic father. Hoffman convinced the German pharmaceutical company he worked for to consider marketing the synthesized version of white willow bark. They began to sell it to pharmacists in a powder form. By 1918 the American firm Sterling Products Inc. bought the rights to trademark the synthesized white willow bark from the German company, Friedrich Bayer. They found a way to mass produce the medicine in tablet form. It became the most widely used drug in the world, and currently 20 billion tablets of aspirin per year are being sold.[3] Every grocery store and pharmacy sells aspirin. Health food stores sell white willow bark. Both are effective painkillers.

The effectiveness of different natural medicines varies. This is a field of medicine which is unregulated, even though the level of skill needed to use herbal medicines safely and effectively is equal to that needed to prescribe synthetic medicines. As a consequence, it's more difficult for a consumer to check the credentials of a specialist in herbs. This is where you have to use good judgment and inform yourself. You can learn about natural and herbal cures in books on the topic. Check your local library and health food stores. If you're interested in learning how to use herbs, vitamins, or nutrition in the prevention and treatment of illnesses, find a book by a reputable author. Once you've informed yourself, you'll be able to make wise decisions for yourself and your family.

Supplements

Changes in FDA regulations in 1994 have resulted in the supplement industry becoming largely unregulated.[4] This means that claims on labels may or may not be true, the quantity of the active ingredient isn't being verified by an independent source, and the FDA doesn't verify product safety.

Literature about a single supplement is not a reliable source of information. The manufacturer of the supplement is likely to have produced such literature, and it's designed to sell the product. Check with outside sources to verify what you learn in sales literature. Books that discuss the properties of many herbs or vitamins are more likely to provide information, not a sales pitch.

Many companies use testimonials to convince you their product is effective. Testimonials are interesting, but they're not good science. You need to know from a source with no interest in the product how a substance brings healing. Remember, literature provided by a manufacturer is always designed to sell the product.

If it seems to you that a supplement promises too much, it probably does. Most herbs and supplements are able to do one or two things, not cure every disease. When people get tricked into buying a useless product, they're less likely to try one that really is effective.

Some supplements have a single characteristic with multiple beneficial consequences. For example, antioxidants provide a general benefit by reducing toxins in the body. The antioxidant vitamin C helps the body repair cells. Since cells are damaged by most diseases or injuries, it's useful in many situations.

Some people mistakenly believe that because an herb is natural, it can't be dangerous. Medicinal herbs are medicines, and they need to be taken appropriately. They shouldn't be randomly sampled, any more than you would randomly try over-the-counter medicines at the drugstore. Do not use herbs until you understand their purpose and know how to take them. Make sure you're being advised by a reliable source, not a salesperson.

Vitamins and minerals are essential to the functioning of the body. Severe deficiencies in vitamins or minerals can have serious health consequences, such as scurvy or rickets. The impact of a moderate or mild deficiency is not as well researched or understood. Scientists do not agree on the optimal amount of vitamins and minerals we need or whether our diet provides adequate quantities.

Theoretically, the vitamins and minerals we need to stay healthy are provided through our food. But there must be sufficient nutrients in the soil where crops are grown to get the optimum benefits. Planting the same crop year after year can deplete the soil of certain nutrients, and the extensive use of chemical fertilizers and pesticides is often used in place of proper soil management, resulting in foods with lower nutritive values.

A diet high in processed foods or junk foods is probably not providing adequate nutrients. As our bodies are confronted with more toxins in the environment, more antioxidants are needed. For these reasons, many people choose to supplement their diet with vitamins.

A multivitamin is a combination of vitamins. Most experts agree that multivitamins are beneficial, but not all multivitamins are the same. This is another situation of "Buyer beware." Some vitamins are derived from natural food sources; others are derived synthetically. The body may not be able to extract the needed vitamins and minerals from every formulation, or it may be more difficult for the body to break down a tablet than a capsule. Some of the brands available for children include dyes and artificial flavors such as NutraSweet.

An informed consumer will want to learn which companies provide the best vitamin products. The better quality brands are generally sold through health food stores. The bottle will usually state that the product contains no dyes, artificial colors, artificial flavors, or preservatives. However, just because a brand is sold in a health food store doesn't mean everything in the product line is good for you.

Supplements are big industry. The sale of vitamins, minerals, herbs, enzymes, amino acids, and natural healing substances generate big profits for an industry that is unregulated, which means that excellent products can be side by side with useless or harmful ones. Many supplements are sold by individual distributors who are convinced the product is helpful but may not know what it does. It's not wise to assume that all the information provided is accurate. Try to learn about the benefits of the product from an objective, independent source.

DENTISTRY

Dentistry is a medical specialty that has excelled in preventive care. Teaching people about brushing their teeth and regular checkups has led to more people maintaining their teeth throughout their lifetime. Dentists are not trained, however, in neurotoxicity. For this reason you will want to make your own decisions about the neurotoxic risks of the following items.

Some dentists recommend artificial sweeteners, such as NutraSweet, in place of sugar to prevent cavities. This is not the official position of the American Dental Association (ADA), because they do not endorse any specific artificial sweetener. The neurotoxicity of NutraSweet is discussed in chapter 13.

The ADA does endorse the use of fluoride, despite the lack of scientific evidence that it actually prevents tooth decay. Increasing numbers of scientific studies are finding that fluoride accumulates in bone and can lead to joint pain, increased risk of fractures, and bone deformation. Fluoride is discussed in chapter 18.

The greatest risk of neurotoxicity from dentistry is the use of mercury. Silver amalgam fillings are composed of about 50 percent mercury. Mercury is a heavy metal, and its poisonous effects are well known. The study of the toxic effects of mercury began over 150 years ago when Tanquerel des Planches studied mirror factory workers in France who began showing neurotoxic symptoms from mercury exposure. Outbreaks of mercury poisonings is Minimata, Japan and in Iraq clearly demonstrated the ability of mercury to cross the placenta and permanently damage a developing baby.[5] The use of mercury in dental offices poses a significant risk to pregnant hygienists, dentists, and assistants.[6]

Scientific studies have shown that after mercury fillings are installed, they continually release minute amounts of mercury vapors. The amount of vapors released after chewing is fifteen times the amount released when the jaw is at rest.[7] Mercury has been shown to accumulate in the brains of humans with mercury fillings.[8]

When mercury fillings were placed in the teeth of a female sheep and the sheep was checked twenty-nine days later, mercury was found in the ewe's blood, urine, feces, muscles, kidney, liver, brain and endocrine glands (pituitary, thyroid, adrenal, pancreas, and ovary).[9]

The controversy over mercury fillings is not new. In 1840 the American Society of Dental Surgeons was formed. Their members were required to sign a pledge promising not to use silver-mercury fillings due to the risk of mercury poisoning. In 1859 the American Dental Association (ADA) was formed. The ADA supported the use of silver-mercury amalgams.[10] Today, the International Association of Oral Medicine and Toxicology, the American Society of Biological Dentistry, and the Wholistic Dental Association continue to oppose the use of silver-mercury amalgams.

Many people have reported neurotoxic symptoms from mercury fillings. The extent to which mercury fillings have caused or contributed to neurodegenerative diseases such as Alzheimer's disease and Parkinson's disease is unknown. If you need to have dental work, avoid silver-mercury fillings. Also avoid the use of other heavy metals in your mouth, such as nickel and copper. Alternatives range from a low-cost composite to high quality gold. Composites are often preferred for fillings because they match the color of your teeth.

PREVENTION

There are two components to prevention. The first is to protect yourself from harm; the second is to strengthen your body. By protecting yourself from neurotoxins, you protect yourself from a chemical injury. To strengthen your body, you will need to live a healthy lifestyle. This includes exercise, a healthy diet, adequate sleep, and antioxidant vitamins or supplements. A healthy lifestyle, which increases your body's strength and resistance to disease, will make you less likely to need medical intervention of any kind.

CHAPTER FIFTEEN

REDUCING TOXINS IN THE GARAGE

There is no regulatory agency to protect you in your garage, so you need to act as your own safety inspector. You can reduce toxic exposures in the garage by purchasing less toxic products, by using toxic products in the safest manner possible, and by proper disposal of hazardous waste.

PURCHASING LESS TOXIC AND NONTOXIC PRODUCTS

In many homes, the garage is a storeroom for old chemicals. Among the toxins found in many garages are pesticides, herbicides, paint products, gasoline, and automotive products. The use of nontoxic pest control and organic lawn and garden techniques will eliminate the need for some of these poisons. Less toxic paint products are also readily available, so this source of toxins can also be replaced. The use of water-based paints eliminates the need for the toxic, solvent-based paint thinners used with oil-based paints. Low-toxicity paints which do not contain volatile organic compounds are discussed in chapter 17.

When selecting varnishes and other types of coatings, water-based solutions will be less toxic than oil-based or solvent-based formulas. Less toxic products are likely to be advertised as environmentally friendly products. When you are selecting materials used for building or art projects, look for less toxic or nontoxic alternatives. If your local hardware store does not provide information about less toxic products, you can turn to the local library for more information. No matter what you are creating, there are non-neurotoxic products you can use. The more knowledgeable someone is about a skill or craft, the more likely he or she is to know about alternative ways to create the project without depending on petrochemicals. If finding the materials you need is difficult in your city, you may want to use mail-order catalogs.

A primary source of toxic fumes in many garages is gasoline fumes from lawnmowers. Gasoline powered lawnmowers are a significant source of air pollution, and you may want to consider using a push mower or one that is electric or solar-powered. If you have to store gasoline in your garage, be sure it's in a tightly sealed, clearly marked container. If you can smell the gas fumes, you may want to use a more airtight container or seal it in a plastic bag.

Automotive products are another significant source of toxins in the garage. Sometimes there are no alternatives that are less toxic, so these chemicals need to be carefully stored and used properly with good ventilation.

HOW TO REDUCE YOUR EXPOSURE WHEN USING TOXIC CHEMICALS

If you left your car running inside a sealed garage, it could be fatal, but the fumes do not accumulate to a fatal level on the open road. When you can't avoid using toxic chemicals, consider ways to increase ventilation to dilute toxic fumes. Consider the airflow patterns in your garage. Are you able to get cross-ventilation? If the only exterior opening is the garage door, you may want to use a large fan to blow out fumes. If your garage opens into your house, you will need to set up a ventilation pattern that doesn't blow chemicals into your home. When a garage is attached to a home, toxic fumes in the garage can seep into the house through the wall or enter the house each time the door between the garage and home is opened. If you use toxic chemicals regularly, you may want to consider using them in a detached building to protect your home.

When you use chemicals, it's important to follow the precautions listed. If gloves or goggles are recommended, there's a good reason. Precautions are not listed unless there is risk of serious injury or other people have already been injured.

One simple safety precaution, which can dramatically reduce your exposure to neurotoxins, is never to use gasoline, acetone, or paint thinner on your skin to remove greasy dirt. These substances quickly penetrate the skin and enter the bloodstream. (If you are trying to convince someone else in your home to end this dangerous practice, you might want to mention that among other risks, exposure to these neurotoxins can lead to sterility or impotence.) Oily, greasy dirt can be removed with another greasy substance. Lard or vegetable oil will remove the greasy dirt, and soap and water will remove the vegetable oil or lard. There are also several products sold in hardware stores specifically for cleaning greasy dirt from your hands.

Another safety precaution when using toxic substances is to shower immediately after you've finished to wash off the chemicals from your skin and hair. Since the residue could also be in your clothing, you may want to put clothes directly into the washing machine so that neither you nor anyone else will have to handle them again. Pregnant women in particular should avoid handling neurotoxic chemicals or clothes with neurotoxic residues.

DISPOSING OF TOXIC PRODUCTS

If you look around your garage, you may find toxic chemical products you want to get rid of. If you are disposing of old paints, pesticides, and herbicides, consult with your city government about safe disposal practices. Be sure to follow the guidelines set by your city to protect your community from toxic waste. Do not simply throw hazardous products into the trash, because they can cause injury to waste management personnel, or they can combine with other toxic waste to produce an even more toxic combination. Throwing toxic products down the drain can contaminate the water supply of your entire city.

If you live outside of a city, you still need to dispose of hazardous materials in a safe manner. Dumping toxins on your property creates a health hazard for you, your family, and future generations. Toxic dumps are often discovered by children as they play. Although proper disposal may be inconvenient or cost a fee, it is your responsibility to ensure safe disposal of the product you bought. In the future, you can make more informed decisions about buying products that do not require toxic waste management.

Be sure to recycle waste oil, brake fluid, transmission fluid, and car batteries. Your local city government can provide information about recycling or proper disposal of these products in your city.

◆◆◆

Toxic chemicals are a health hazard during their production, use, and disposal. The solution to toxic waste management is to reduce toxic waste production. As consumers, we can choose to use less-toxic or nontoxic products, which will eventually cause companies to produce safer and more beneficial products in place of harmful ones. When you make wise choices about the products you buy, you're protecting your health, your family's health, and the health of your community.

CHAPTER SIXTEEN

NONTOXIC LAWNS AND GARDENS

The production of herbicides is the fastest growing part of the pesticide industry.[1] Herbicides are neurotoxic in their own right, and their production yields an even more dangerous byproduct, dioxin. Dioxin is one of the most toxic substances known to man and is known to cause tumors and birth defects at very low concentrations.[2]

Agent Orange —2,4,5-Trichlorophenoxyacetic acid, (2,4,5-T), 2,4-dichlorophenoxyacetl acid (2,4-D), and traces of dioxin— is the most infamous of the herbicides. It was used in Vietnam to defoliate the jungles. The injuries to American soldiers caused by Agent Orange resulted in the largest personal injury suit in history up to that time.[3]

How does that relate to civilian life where herbicides sold for home use are not as potent as Agent Orange? The Vietnam soldiers were not exposed to Agent Orange on a daily basis while playing on swings, making mud pies, running across the yard, or chewing on sticks and leaves. No child or pet should be exposed to these toxic chemicals in their own yard.

Herbicides do not stay where they're put. They travel by water and by air. Rainwater washes herbicides off yards and fields into groundwater sources. In dry weather, the toxic particles are blown by the wind and sometimes carried great distances. Toxic particles come back to earth when winds shift or rain carries them down. The herbicide alachlor has been detected in rainwater at levels up to 6.59 ppb. By 1988, herbicides and insecticides were detected in the groundwater of twenty-six states.[4]

Any word that ends in *-cide* refers to killing—homicide, suicide, pesticide, insecticide, herbicide, fungicide, termiticide. So it shouldn't surprise you that herbicides—the chemicals of death—will not foster plant life.

If you're controlling your yard or garden with neurotoxic chemicals, you're inadvertently destroying the natural environmental balance. This can lead to more diseased plants, weeds, and an onslaught of pests.

Herbicides kill important and beneficial creatures you want in your yard or garden, such as earthworms, honeybees, and microorganisms. Earthworms loosen and aerate the soil, which facilitates plant growth. Honeybees pollinate plants. The destruction of honeybee populations costs agriculture $135 million each year because of reduced crop yields and lost honey.[5] Microorganisms, such as bacteria and fungi, feed your plants by decomposing sugars, complex carbohydrates, and proteins in organic matter, and they release minerals when they die. The functioning of these microscopic creatures is so complex that scientists are just beginning to learn how to work with, rather than against, their natural processes.[6]

In addition to altering the biological system that facilitates plant growth, herbicides and insecticides destroy important natural defenses against insects. Bird and bat populations have been decreased by pesticide use.[7] Bats consume about a third of their weight every night in moths, beetles, mosquitoes, flies, grasshoppers, cockroaches, termites, flying ants, and other insects. Pesticide use has reduced the bat population at Carlsbad Caverns, New Mexico, for example, from approximately 8.7 million in 1936 to 218,000 in 1973.[8]

After the application of pesticides, pest populations can increase because their natural predators are destroyed. Target pests often develop resistance to insecticides and herbicides, whereas their predators do not. More than 440 insects and mite species and 70 fungus species are known to be resistant to some pesticides.[9]

Destroying a pest population is not always in our best interest. Sometimes a secondary pest gets out of control because the primary pest is not there to eat it. For example, in 1900 the major pests which attacked cotton were the boll weevil and the cotton leaf worm. Now that pesticides have been used extensively, the cotton bollworm, tobacco budworm, cotton aphid, and spider mite have all become serious threats. In California, twenty-four of the top twenty-five agricultural pests are secondary pests.[10]

Herbicides and insecticides threaten our water supplies, they destroy beneficial insects, and they damage communities of beneficial microorganisms. Using chemicals on a yard or garden destroys the natural ecosystem and threatens the health of your family and your neighbors. In a cost/benefit analysis, the cost of herbicides in human health and plant loss are high. The benefits of herbicides appear to be only for the companies that sell them.

LAWNS

One way to improve the health of your lawn is to use a lawn mower with a mulching blade and leave the grass clippings on the lawn to provide nourishment. You can also assist the microorganisms in your flower beds and around your shrubs by adding a layer of mulch to protect them from the sun.

If your lawn needs additional fertilizer, be sure that the fertilizer is made from a natural source such as earthworm castings, bat guano, blood meal, bone meal, chicken by-products, or steer manure. A chemical fertilizer will overstimulate and eventually kill the microorganisms in the soil. The overstimulation of the microorganisms causes chemically treated lawns to be very green.

This unnatural effect can be compared to what happens to an athlete who abuses steroids. Steroids are man-made hormones that cause muscles to grow at an unnatural rate. While this may look good, it is harmful to the body. The muscles developed by steroids are prone to injury because the tendons and ligaments have not developed at the same rate. (Some of the side effects of steroid hormone abuse include altered secondary sex characteristics, personality changes, and cancer.) Steroid use can help an athlete win a game, but it can destroy his life.

In a similar manner, chemical lawn treatments can make a lawn look good for a season, but in the long run they will weaken the ecosystem the lawn depends on for life.

Many people hire companies to manage their lawns chemically. You shouldn't have to risk your health to have a lovely lawn just because you prefer to have someone else take care of it for you. One nontoxic option is to hire an individual or lawn care company that doesn't use toxic chemicals.

You will want to ask the company how they will care for your lawn. Just because they claim to use "organic" methods doesn't mean they do. Legitimate organic lawn care will focus on improving the health of your soil in order to increase the health of the plants so they can resist pests, weeds, and diseases. Often changes in mowing and watering patterns, aerating, reducing thatch, fertilizing, and balancing the soil pH will improve the health of a lawn.[11]

Lawn care companies that depend on chemical treatments may recommend pre-emergent herbicides to prevent seeds from germinating. While this does prevent some weeds, it also kills the microorganisms in the soil. This causes lifeless, unhealthy soil which will be vulnerable to future weeds and pests.

Herbicides are often used to kill dandelions and other broadleaf plants. Ironically, herbicides can make a lawn more susceptible to all kinds of weeds and pests. Instead of using an herbicide, you can remove dandelions manually before they spread their seeds. A thick, healthy lawn will prevent dandelions and other weeds from sprouting.

When a yard has been heavily treated with chemicals, it takes time for the natural ecosystem to rebuild, sometimes a couple of years. The ground is ill if the microorganisms and beneficial pests have been destroyed, and it will take time for them to return. But if they're given a chance, they will return. The T-shirt slogan "Get your lawn off drugs!" may be the best advice.

When the soil recovers, the lawn may grow back better and stronger than ever. A healthy ecosystem leads to healthy grass that is able to resist weed and insect infestations.[12]

If your lawn or garden has serious problems, you may want to hire a horticulture consultant, lawn consultant, or ornamental horticulturist. Find out before you hire someone whether they are committed to helping you find natural solutions, rather than depending on neurotoxic chemicals.

Many health food stores carry natural lawn products. Safer Company makes low toxicity weed killers with natural substances and natural pyrethrums. You can create a deadly weed killer that is safe for people by combining a tablespoon of soap in a gallon of vinegar. This mixture will kill any plant it touches, particularly in hot weather, so apply it carefully. This is an excellent way to kill weeds that grow in cracks in the cement.[13]

PLANTS AND GARDENS

A wealth of information about organic gardening is available in bookstores and public libraries, as well as in magazines devoted to the subject. Some magazines not only provide useful information, they allow gardeners to share their successes with one another. In one such magazine, a reader wrote about her success with using powdered milk as a fertilizer for her flowers.[14] Many organic gardening books have reference sections about how to handle a specific pest. For example, infestations of aphids and spider mites can be controlled by spraying the plant with soapy water in place of a neurotoxic insecticide.[15]

Organic gardening books are likely to focus on increasing the health of your soil, selecting appropriate plants for your location and amount of shade, and picking healthy plants at the outset. Many plants defend themselves by triggering pest-repelling chemicals.[16] Insects and diseases usually attack plants that are already sick, so increasing the health of the plants enables them to resist their predators naturally.

Healthy soil is important in growing healthy vegetables and flowers. The nutrients plants need from soil include nitrogen, phosphorus, and potassium. These nutrients can come from natural sources, including certain plants. In place of chemical fertilizers, for example, planting legumes provides a natural source of nitrogen.[17]

If there is a fungus on your plants, you do not have to use a neurotoxic chemical fungicide to treat them. As you may remember from chapter 13, 90 percent of chemical fungicides have been found to cause tumors in laboratory animals.[18] A natural alternative is to alter the acidity of the plant with a mixture of four teaspoons of baking soda per gallon of water. Apply this solution only to the plant (such as a rose bush) or turf you are treating, being careful not to spill it onto soil you do not want to treat.[19]

～

The destructive power of herbicides and insecticides affect life forms as small as a fungi and as large as a human. They destroy natural biological systems and natural pest controls. In the process, they make a yard or garden increasingly dependent on toxic chemicals.

Plants are part of a living system, and the care they need should promote life, not death! In the midst of all the pollution and destruction in the world, your yard can be a sanctuary of life where plants, animals, and humans can flourish.

4 teaspoons baking soda
per gallon of H_2O.

CHAPTER SEVENTEEN

LOW-TOXICITY HOME IMPROVEMENT AND CONSTRUCTION

Air is so basic to our existence that it's easy to take it for granted. Yet the air we breathe has a profound effect on our health and well-being.

When NASA was preparing to send astronauts into space, they found that astronauts were getting "space flu" from the spacecraft, so NASA began to investigate the problem. They found that materials used in the spacecraft were emitting toxic fumes. These materials posed a considerable risk to astronauts trapped in a small space without any opportunity for an exchange of air. With this finding, NASA created an inventory of the amount and type of chemicals emitted by their materials.[1] This list helps guide them in selecting more appropriate materials.

The more we seal up and insulate our homes and offices to conserve energy, the more they resemble the spacecraft. Sick building syndrome is an earthbound version of space flu. It's primarily caused by tightly sealed office buildings without an adequate exchange of fresh air. When remodeling occurs in these buildings, the solvents, formaldehyde, and other toxic fumes are sealed in the air supply, and people can be injured by the neurotoxins emitted. Sometimes the toxins are generated by work activities inside the building. Hospitals, for example, generate numerous neurotoxic chemicals. If these chemicals are not vented to the outside, they can recirculate throughout the building. Standard offices need to have outside venting to eliminate the chemicals used in photocopying.

Toxic building conditions can also exist in a home. When toxic materials are used in the construction of a home, they contaminate the air by outgassing. The terms *emission* and *outgassing* refer to the fumes emitted by a material. Sometimes these fumes can be detected because of their odor. For example, that "new car smell" is caused by chemicals outgassing from the car interior. The smell of new paint or new carpeting is also caused by outgassing. In addition to being unpleasant, these fumes can contain neurotoxic chemicals.

Many of the sources of indoor air pollution have already been addressed in this book: neurotoxic pesticides, housecleaning chemicals, and synthetic fragrances. Other products that can contribute to indoor air pollution are building materials, carpeting, paint, furnishings, and natural gas.

BUILDING MATERIALS

The best way to avoid toxic emissions is to use less-toxic and nontoxic products from the beginning. When building a new home or remodeling an existing structure, it is important to select materials with the lowest emissions rate. Neurotoxic chemicals to avoid are formaldehyde and petroleum-based solvents, such as toluene, xylene, benzene compounds, and acetone. The Materials Safety Data Sheets (MSDS), the NASA ranking of materials, EPA publications, and books on the subject of nontoxic construction practices are all sources of information about construction materials.

Hard materials such as stone, cement, ceramic, or steel have low emission rates, whereas foam, soft plastics, and plywood have higher emission rates. Consider the products used in each stage of construction.

Floors
In flooring, select a low-emission material like ceramic tile, brick, concrete, hardwood, or cork-based linoleum. Linoleum is made largely of natural materials, whereas vinyl composition flooring is

likely to outgas hydrocarbons. Pay attention to the adhesives used. Water-based adhesives are less toxic than solvent-based adhesives. Adhesives should not contain formaldehyde or neurotoxic solvents such as toluene, xylene, benzene, ketones, and acetone.

Insulation

You can compare the amount of formaldehyde used in different fiberglass insulations by consulting the Materials Safety Data Sheet, which should be available from the company selling the insulation. Urea formaldehyde should never be used for insulation. Urea formaldehyde foam insulation, or UFFI, releases measurable amounts of formaldehyde gas for a prolonged period of time.[2] Due to the number of chemical injuries caused by urea formaldehyde insulation, it was banned for use on homes. Even if this ban is lifted, however, this product should never be used.

Ventilation

When designing a home or office, be sure to consider ventilation. Well-placed windows that open to the outside allow for a good exchange of fresh air, which will prevent a space flu type of condition. Strategically placed windows can also reduce the need for air-conditioning.

After construction, allow time to ventilate so the materials can outgas before people inhabit the building. An indication of outgassing is "new building smell." You can increase the rate of outgassing by heating the building and then opening all the windows to let the fumes escape. No one should be in the building while it is heated.

Pressedwood Products

Particleboard is made from wood shavings compressed and held together with a urea-formaldehyde resin. Plywood is several sheets of wood sandwiched together with a phenol-formaldehyde resin. Both of these products release low levels of formaldehyde.[3]

Prefabricated housing is often made of particleboard, and there have been cases of chemical injuries caused by high levels of formaldehyde from these structures. A pungent odor can sometimes alert you to the presence of formaldehyde. If you suspect that a health symptom is related to a prefabricated building, see if the symptom disappears if you are away from the building for several days. If a child complains about headaches or difficulties thinking in classes located in prefabricated buildings, it may be due to formaldehyde. An environmental engineer or an industrial hygienist should be able to measure formaldehyde levels.

CARPETS

Hundreds of chemicals can outgas from carpeting, particularly if the carpet is defective. One of the toxic by-products of the latex backing is 4-phenylcyclohexene (4-PC), a powerful neurotoxin which is structurally similar to phencyclidine. Phencyclidine is well-known for its ability to alter brain functioning; in everyday language it's known as angel dust.[4] Select a carpet without a latex backing to reduce this source of toxicity in the carpet. It's especially important to prevent toxic emissions when you have young children crawling around on the floor.

If you're planning to install carpet, you'll be on your own in selecting one low in neurotoxins. The "green label" on carpets is an industry gimmick and does not guarantee a low-toxicity product.

To select low-toxicity carpeting, look for 100 percent nylon fiber woven into the backing without a secondary backing. The colorful carpeting fibers should be stuck directly into a tough, burlap-appearing backing without any type of adhesive or latex material glued to it.

If the carpet is advertised as stain-resistant, it's been chemically treated. If you can smell any type of adhesive or dye, look for another type. Ask for a sample of the carpet and see if you can smell it when you take it out of the store (if you don't have a good sense of smell, check with someone who does). You can find out from the manufacturer if the carpet has been treated with an "antimicrobial" agent, which is a pesticide.

After selecting low-toxicity carpet, you will need to consider the carpet pad, which is also a potential source of neurotoxins. Carpet pads can contain almost anything. Due to the instability of this industry, there are no regulations or standards. The best alternative is not to use a pad at all.

Carpet installation is another potential source of injury, since carpet glues outgas neurotoxins. (Glue-sniffing is a well-known method of getting high and causing brain damage.) No one needs to inhale toxic fumes in their own home, so install carpet by manually tacking or stapling it, rather than using glue.

If defective carpeting has been installed, it's a health hazard that needs to be taken seriously. How do you know if you have defective carpeting? You may notice indoor plants turning black or brown, dead insects, and health problems in pets and people. If the carpeting continues to have a strong odor after the first month, it's possible it could be a chemically contaminated batch. If anyone is experiencing symptoms that show up while being around the new carpeting but dissipate when away from the carpeting, the carpet may be a hazard.

A less risky alternative to carpeting is tile, linoleum, concrete, or hardwood flooring, using cotton or wool rugs without toxic adhesives.

PAINT

Everyone has experienced the noxious odor of freshly applied paint. In addition to being unpleasant, these fumes can contain any of 300 toxic chemicals,[5] including the neurotoxic solvents trichloroethylene, benzene, toluene, xylene, and ketones. Fortunately for consumers, some pioneers in the paint industry are selling paints that do not contain volatile organic compounds (VOCs). These low-toxicity paints are available from major distributors, so it doesn't make sense to use anything else in a home or office. At the time of writing this book, Glidden 2000 and Benjamin Moore Pristine are no-VOC paints available through national distribution centers. There are also specialty companies that produce less toxic and nontoxic paints. You can even make your own paint from whitewash or a milk base.[6]

If you're preparing a room for a new baby, be sure to use the least toxic materials available. After preparing the room, thoroughly ventilate it. You can heat the room to increase the rate of outgassing and then ventilate again.

Community organizations, such as churches, senior citizens' centers, and volunteer organizations need to use no-VOC paint and safe building materials to protect the people they're trying to serve. School districts and day-care centers should make it a priority to use low-toxicity and nontoxic materials around children.

In a business setting, it makes good financial sense to use no-VOC paints. Both customers and employees are going to be more comfortable in an office without toxic, noxious paint fumes, and employees are likely to be more productive.

Sometimes you can't control the type of paint that has been applied, particularly when moving into a home or an apartment. In this situation, you can facilitate the outgassing and drying process by increasing ventilation and by heating the room and then opening the windows to let the fumes escape. The paint-contaminated air inside the home or business needs to be exchanged with fresh, outside air. If the windows do not open, prop open the door.

Another way to reduce paint fumes is to fill a large bowl with baking soda or white vinegar, which will slowly absorb the paint odors. Vinegar is particularly effective in closets that have a persistent paint odor. A more powerful way to draw in paint fumes is with a molecular adsorber. This nontoxic device is filled with very dry particles that attract chemical-laden water molecules (see appendix A).

A chemical air freshener is not a wise way to manage paint fumes; it just adds a second source of neurotoxic pollution.

FURNISHINGS

It is important to select less-toxic and nontoxic furnishings for your home. Pressedwood products (particle board and plywood) are often used in furniture, particularly inexpensive furnishings. To check for hidden particleboard, look underneath furniture before purchasing it to see if the particleboard is visible. There will be less formaldehyde outgassing if the particleboard is old or completely covered by some type of laminate. It's best to select furniture at the outset that doesn't contain pressedwood products. You will particularly want to avoid pressedwood products around your bed, where you will be exposed to it for an extended period of time. When you can't avoid particleboard (in kitchen cabinets, for instance), you may want to cover it with a nontoxic sealant or paint.

The fabrics and fibers used on sofas and stuffed chairs are often petrochemical products, such as polyesters and foams. You will particularly want to avoid fabric that has been chemically treated. Check to see if a particular piece of furniture has a strong odor before you purchase it, because this could indicate a higher rate of emissions. If you do purchase new furniture, keep it in a well ventilated room while it is new and is emitting chemicals at a higher rate. Older furniture is less likely to emit neurotoxins.

To select less toxic and nontoxic furniture, look for real wood, metal, cotton fabric, cotton stuffing, and glass. You may also want to consider the types of paints, varnishes, and sealants used on the product, although most dried coatings do not continue to emit neurotoxins.

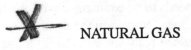 NATURAL GAS

Another contributor to indoor air pollution is the emissions from natural gas appliances. If you use gas appliances in your home, it's critical that the gas combustion products are properly vented to the outside to prevent carbon monoxide and other neurotoxins from accumulating inside your house. A leaky furnace can release lethal levels of carbon monoxide. You can purchase carbon monoxide detectors, which work like smoke detectors to warn you of danger.

A sealed furnace system should not be emitting hydrocarbons into your home if it functions properly. If you ever smell gas fumes, have the gas company come out immediately to check for a leak. Also, schedule annual maintenance service. It's imperative that gas appliances and furnaces function at peak efficiency.

Although some modern appliances have decreased the toxicity of gas power, all-electric homes eliminate this source of chronic, low-level neurotoxicity. If you are looking for a new home, you may want to consider one that is all electric.

∽

Sometimes it takes extra effort to locate and use low-toxicity products, but the effort is well worth it when you consider that you're protecting the air you and your family will breathe, perhaps for years into the future.

CHAPTER EIGHTEEN

AIR AND WATER FILTERS

In 1992, U.S. companies reported to the EPA that they released 1.84 billion pounds of toxic chemicals into the air.[1] This figure doesn't include illegal dumping releases in Mexico or Canada, or ground and water pollution. Air pollution is a serious health threat. A full explanation of all the pollutants in our nation's air, however, is beyond the scope of this book. If you're interested in a hair-raising description of air pollution, read *The Toxic Cloud* by Michael Brown.[2]

What most people want to know is whether or not they need an air filter (or water filter) system. Often the people who advocate using filters are selling them, so you might wonder about their motives. This chapter will attempt to provide objective information about air and water filters. Whether or not you and your family need to purchase filter systems will depend on your current health and the level of pollution where you live.

AIR FILTRATION

Electrostatic Filters

Every home with central air can benefit from using an electrostatic filter, which replaces the standard fiberglass filters used with furnaces and air-conditioning systems. Electrostatic filters depend on the power of static cling to trap dust, pollen, and mold particles. These filters are usually made of hard plastic fibers or foams. As particles go through the materials, they rub against the fiber and develop static electricity. The first layer of dust attracts the next layer. Static cling holds the dust in the filter the way it holds a sock to a sweater in your dryer. An electrostatic filter will visibly reduce the amount of dust in a home, which will reduce the need for housecleaning.

The filter should be wiped off or hosed down about once a month. Sturdier filters will last longer; some are guaranteed for five years. Be sure the mesh is tightly woven so it's effective. Electrostatic filters of different quality grades are sold in most hardware stores. Top-quality filters are sold by companies that sell air-purifying equipment.

Sometimes people combine an air-duct cleaning with purchase of an electrostatic filter. If you have your air ducts cleaned, be sure the company doesn't use chemicals to clean or to prevent future mold growth. The neurotoxic chemicals in the fungicide (mold killer) could be more harmful than the mold.

Charcoal Filters
A charcoal filter medium is used in an air filter to remove neurotoxic chemicals. This type of filter becomes important if your home is susceptible to chemical pollution. Some parts of the country are so polluted that every home in the area would benefit from an air-filtering system. Homes located near an industry that releases toxic emissions, such as a chemical or petroleum manufacturer, should be equipped with good quality air filters. A home next door to a gas station, dry cleaner, print shop, autobody and paint business, or other business that uses high levels of neurotoxic chemicals would benefit from an air-filtering system, as would a home located next to a freeway or major road where pollution is high from exhaust fumes containing carbon monoxide, lead, benzene, and other neurotoxins.

If someone in your home has allergies, asthma, repeated infections, hyperactivity, fatigue, or symptoms of neurotoxicity, the investment in an air filter can be an important medical decision. Selecting an appropriate air filter is like selecting other home appliances—it's a serious investment. Although it may seem expensive, if it reduces illness and health-care costs, it's a great value. From the perspective of reducing neurotoxic chemicals, a low-quality filter will probably be of no value at all.

Charcoal is the filtering medium used to filter neurotoxic chemicals. If a different material is being used, it's not filtering neurotoxins. Although numerous types of filters are made, few companies specialize in the removal of neurotoxic chemicals. Appendix A lists two companies I'm aware of that offer filters that successfully remove neurotoxins from the air. If you select a filter from a different company, be sure the filter is actually improving the quality of the air. Beware of plastic housing—heated plastic can emit toxins. Check the air coming out of the filter. It should smell clean, and you should not be able to detect a chemical residue. Be sure that over time the air continues to smell clean, because a poorly designed motor can outgas after it becomes hot, which will re-contaminate the filtered air.

For homes with central air, a combination electrostatic/charcoal filter panel can filter the entire home. For most people, this is the best value. The panel filter is used in place of the standard fiberglass furnace filter. The charcoal portion filters neurotoxins and the electrostatic portion filters dusts, molds, and pollens. It uses the power of the air system in the house to pull air through it, so you don't pay for a motorized filter unit.

A quality portable, free-standing charcoal filter may cost between $200 and $400. A combination electrostatic/charcoal panel filter is available for about half the cost of a free-standing unit.

WATER POLLUTION

Water pollution in this country is widespread. Every year companies release millions of pounds of toxic waste into water. In 1992 alone, companies reported to the EPA that 273 million pounds of toxic waste were released into surface water. Water supplies were further threatened that year by 338 million pounds of toxic waste on land and 726 million pounds of toxic waste legally injected underground.[3] The amount of water contamination from illegal dumping by industries and individuals is unknown.

Contaminants from agriculture also threaten surface water. Rainwater and flooding carry pesticide residues into streams and rivers. In addition to traveling by water, contaminants can travel airborne for enormous distances. Scientists are beginning to appreciate the mobility of neurotoxic chemicals after finding chlorinated hydrocarbon pesticides such as toxaphene and chlordane in the Great Lakes. DDT residues may be traveling to the Great Lakes from as far as South America. The herbicide alachlor has been measured in rainwater, which means it was traveling airborne before being rained down to earth.

Groundwater is also vulnerable to chemical contamination. By 1988, pesticides were detected in the groundwater of twenty-six states, and 46 percent of all U.S. counties have groundwater that is susceptible to contamination from agricultural pesticides or fertilizers. The most commonly detected pesticides in groundwater were the herbicide atrazine and the insecticide aldicarb. Aldicarb is the most toxic pesticide registered by the EPA (LD50 0.9 milligrams/kilogram). It's been found in the groundwater of sixteen states.[4]

Additives in Water

Some chemicals, such as chlorine, are intentionally added to city water supplies to kill bacteria and prevent outbreaks of disease. We all know that too much chlorine in water makes it undesirable; nobody wants to drink water that smells like a swimming pool. The amount of chlorine in tap water can accumulate in the body and lead to a chemical injury. Chlorine and its byproducts (including chloroform, trihalomethanes, and nonvolatile chlorinated hydrocarbons) can increase rates of bladder cancer, colon cancer, and rectum cancer.[5] Chlorine also interacts with organic matter in the water to generate additional chemical compounds.

Approximately half of U.S. water systems add another chemical into their water supplies—fluoride. Most of us grew up thinking of fluoride as a healthy way to keep our teeth strong and cavity-free. In fact, the use of fluoride in water systems is the result of one of the greatest sales jobs in history. Fluoride is an industrial waste product, a byproduct of aluminum production and other industries. Currently, the fluoride used for city water systems is the byproduct of phosphate fertilizer manufacturing.

In the 1930s a dentist named Trendley Dean was investigating cases of dental mottling (colored specks on teeth). He found that mottling occurred in communities with natural sources of fluoride. To his surprise, he noticed that people in these communities also seemed to have low levels of tooth decay. He guessed that fluoride might strengthen teeth. For the aluminum industry, which was concerned about lawsuits from people injured by fluoride, it was a golden opportunity. They funded industry scientists to write studies and convince the Public Health Service and the American Dental Association that fluoride would strengthen children's teeth. In a stroke of genius, an industry was able to sell off their toxic waste product and represent it as a benefit.

When fluoride is added to your drinking water, your body stores it in your bones and teeth. (Most toxins are stored in fat cells, but lead and fluoride are deposited in bone.) Fluoride stored in bone slowly accumulates over the years. It can cause a condition called skeletal fluorosis. In its most severe form, skeletal fluorosis leaves a person deformed and crippled. The ligaments calcify, bony spurs appear on limb bones, and the vertebrae partially fuse together.[6]

A mild case of skeletal fluorosis mimics arthritis. There is no way to know how many elderly people are currently diagnosed with arthritis when they actually have skeletal fluorosis caused by a lifetime of fluoride consumption. There is evidence that an accumulation of fluoride can weaken the bones of the elderly, making them more susceptible to bone fractures, particularly hip fractures.[7] A fractured hip or pelvis is a serious concern that can make an elderly person dependent on others. Broken bones are a leading cause of nursing home admissions. For this reason, purified water is an excellent investment in preventive medicine for the elderly.

Fluoride's ability to cause birth defects is unknown. Several studies have shown an increase in cases of Down's syndrome births in fluoridated cities compared to nonfluoridated cities, but these studies were not conclusive.[8] Drinking purified water during pregnancy is especially important, due to all of the potential contaminants in water. A reverse osmosis water filter could be the greatest gift ever given to the new baby. If grandparents or other relatives want to invest in the future, purified water during pregnancy is an excellent gift.

People with any type of kidney dysfunction may be highly vulnerable to the toxic effects of fluoride (as well as other contaminants), and they need to drink filtered water.

Ironically, there is no evidence that fluoride prevents tooth decay. It's true that tooth decay has decreased over the past forty years, but it has decreased in places without fluoridated water as well. Some studies find that areas with fluoridated water have the same rate of tooth decay as areas without fluoridated water, and other studies show that areas with fluoridated water have more tooth decay than areas without fluoridated water. Tooth decay tends to decrease as socioeconomic status increases.[9]

The campaign of misinformation about fluoride was so successful that even today, as more and more scientific evidence demonstrates the toxicity of fluoride, there are professionals who are still convinced that fluoride is beneficial. The American Dental Association continues to advocate the use of fluoride.

In 1986 both the Natural Resources Defense Council and the EPA Union filed a lawsuit against the EPA, charging that scientific evidence about fluoride toxicity was ignored in favor of political goals.[10]

The political battle over fluoride is far from over. In the meantime, you'll want to protect yourself and your family from the known hazards of this chemical.

WATER FILTRATION

Everyone would benefit from drinking pure water. Because of the widespread contamination of our water supplies, the alternatives available to most of us are to purchase purified water or a water purifying system. In the long run, it's more economical to own your own system.

There are three types of water filters available: charcoal filters, water distillers, and reverse osmosis systems. A water softener is not a filter, and it doesn't remove chemicals from water. Water softeners reduce the hardness of the water, often by adding sodium. If you have a water softener, your drinking water will still need to be purified.

Charcoal Filters

At the very least, most homes need a charcoal filter. Charcoal absorbs chlorine and many chemical compounds from water. The more contact the water has with activated charcoal, the more chemicals the charcoal is able to remove.

Activated charcoal filters are widely available. There can be considerable differences in the cost and quality of different systems. Generally, a larger unit is able to provide more contact. The charcoal does need to be replaced at regular intervals.

Distillers

Another method of purifying water is by distillation. These units boil water in one container to create steam. The steam rises and travels to a second container, which should be glass, that collects the steam after it cools and becomes water again. Particles are left behind in the first container. Distillers remove most chemicals from water, except those that boil at the same temperature as water. Distillers do not remove chlorine, so they should be combined with a charcoal filter. A disadvantage of distilled water is that it tastes flat because all the minerals have been removed.

Reverse Osmosis

The best water filtering systems are reverse osmosis (RO). In these units, the water pressure forces water through the reverse osmosis membrane. This membrane separates water at a molecular level. Clean water passes through the membrane into a storage tank and the contaminated water goes down the drain.

A good RO system should have at least three filters. The first filter is a sediment filter that removes large particles from the water. This initial filter protects the membrane from being damaged by larger particles and reduces the amount of filtering the membrane has to do, so it lasts longer. This is important because the RO membrane is the most expensive filter to replace. After the sediment is removed, the water passes through the reverse osmosis membrane. It is then stored in some type of tank until it's used. When you actually fill your glass with water, the water moves from the tank through the third filter, which is a charcoal filter. The charcoal filter is able to remove any residue the water picked up in the storage tank, and it removes the last traces of chlorine. The trace amount of chlorine in the tank prevents any growth of bacteria.

RO water retains trace levels of minerals, which makes it taste good. Since the water tastes good, your family is likely to drink more of it. The money you can save on sodas and drink mixes may help offset the cost of the unit.

If you're filtering well water or water from a nonchlorinated system, add an ultraviolet light to an RO system to prevent bacterial or mold growth. Distilling systems prevent any type of bacterial or mold growth, due to boiling the water. With a charcoal filter, be sure to follow the manufacturer's instructions about replacing charcoal or rinsing it off. Adding a chemical bactericide or fungicide would re-contaminate the water.

When selecting an RO unit, consider the materials used in the filter. Soft plastics can release hydrocarbons into the water (remember, plastic is made from petroleum). Polypropelene is a hard plastic that will not release contaminants, so it's probably the best material available for the tubing. In a well-designed RO system, the water is filtered after being stored, so anything picked up in the tank is removed.

A reverse osmosis unit is a hefty investment, but a good water filter is one appliance people tend to appreciate more and more over time. Generally it will cost between $300 and $700. Some companies lease RO systems, so you don't have to make an up-front investment. The cost of a RO unit may seem high, but the cost of not owning such a system should also be considered. Chemical injuries are more costly than water filters—health care and sick days are expensive, and nursing home care is costly. If removing fluoride from your water can help prevent fractured bones, it's an excellent investment.

There are numerous manufacturers of water systems, and it's worth bargain hunting for a RO system, because the same level of quality can have a wide price range. Companies in your area will be listed in the phone book. Appendix A also lists some mail-order companies.

A reputable dealer will want to answer your questions and help you to be well-informed. If you're being pressured to buy, or if the dealer avoids answering your questions, work with another company.

Pre-Purified Water

If you're not currently in a position to own your own filtering unit, you can purchase purified water. The best value is probably the reverse osmosis water dispensers located at many grocery stores. The cost is reasonable because you provide your own container. Use a glass container, which is the best way to store water. Plastic containers, particularly soft plastics, can emit hydrocarbons back into the water.

There are many companies that sell bottled water. Labels such as "natural water," "spring water," and "mineral water" do not indicate the source of the water or its purity. Unless the company gives you the name of a specific spring, the water is likely to be local tap water that has been filtered.

Whole House Systems

A reverse osmosis system is only appropriate for drinking water. To set up a RO system for an entire house is not feasible. The filtered water could pick up lead, copper, or plastic residues from the pipes inside the house, and there would be too much waste water from the filtering process. Besides, there's no reason to flush your toilet with purified water.

To filter the water in an entire house, a charcoal filtering system should be used. Activated charcoal water filters for the home are available at hardware stores and through specialty dealers. The price of these units will vary, but even a small unit can help reduce the chemicals in your water.

You can also purchase a charcoal filter specifically for your shower if you live in a city with high levels of chlorine in the water. Hot, chlorinated water can release a gas of chloroform, trihalomethanes, and nonvolatile chlorinated hydrocarbons—something you can guard against.

In some places, other toxins are present in the water. For example, one woman noticed that she experienced neurotoxic symptoms after showering. Upon investigation, she found that the water in her city had the second highest rate of PCB contamination in the U.S. As a result, she invested in a top-quality whole house charcoal filtering system to reduce the PCBs.

WATER TESTING

Sometimes people want to know what chemical residues are present in their tap water. Cities generally monitor water for about twenty different chemicals. If there's reason to believe a specific contaminant is in the water, or if there's public outcry, then a city could run an additional test to detect a specific substance. Tests reveal whether the single pollutant tested is present at the time of testing. It doesn't prevent future contamination from illegal dumping, floods washing over farmland and pulling pesticides into water sources, or neurotoxic chemicals traveling in the atmosphere and landing in water supplies.

Laboratory tests analyze your tap water for contaminants. Test batteries begin at $100. The more chemicals tested, the higher the cost. (Remember, over 70,000 chemicals are currently registered with the EPA.) If test results do not reveal chemical residues, you could be given a false sense of security. The lab may not have tested for a particular substance, or the water could be contaminated at a later time. For most people, it makes more sense to invest in a good quality filtering system than to pay for testing. A good system will protect you from contamination now and in the future.

ᑌ

Air and water are necessities of life. We may not be used to having to spend money for them, but it has become increasingly less likely that we can trust the safety of air and water in our homes. It's up to us to protect ourselves.

CHAPTER NINETEEN

MANAGING TOXINS AT WORK

In your home you have a legal right, and the ability, to make changes that will protect you from neurotoxic poisoning. You do not have as much control in a job setting. By paying attention to the use of neurotoxic chemicals at work, however, you can provide extra protection for yourself.

INDUSTRIAL WORK

Numerous neurotoxic chemicals may be used in an industrial work setting. This requires clear safety procedures for working with these chemicals and a Materials Safety Data Sheet (MSDS) provided to workers. It's important to follow the safety precautions designed to protect you from a dangerous or deadly acute exposure. In addition to these precautions, consider ways to reduce your day-to-day exposures so that neurotoxins don't accumulate in your body more rapidly than you're able to detoxify them.

You may want to consider how to avoid breathing chemical fumes. Do you have the option of going outside during your breaks, or avoiding strong cleaning chemicals, or increasing ventilation in your work area? Always use gloves when working with solvents; never let solvents directly touch your skin.

If you work with strong chemicals, you can reduce the number of hours per day you're exposed to residual chemical fumes by showering as soon as you come home and washing your clothes immediately, or storing them in the garage.

If you're working with chemicals known to be neurotoxic, pay attention to your health. If you're becoming irritable, fatigued, disinterested in your family, forgetful, easily angered, uncoordinated, or impotent, it may indicate that your body isn't able to detoxify from the chemical exposures as rapidly as it's being exposed.

Often when a person begins to show personality changes, his or her spouse is the first to notice. Look again at the symptoms listed in chapter 2 and see if they apply to you. If not, use good safety precautions to maintain your health.

If you find you're experiencing neurotoxic symptoms, you can do several things to improve your health. By eliminating neurotoxins from your home and diet, you will reduce your overall level of exposure. Exercise, antioxidant vitamins, and a more nutritious diet may help you increase your body's ability to detoxify. Consult with a nutritionist or a doctor who is trained in the body's nutritional needs, or read about vitamins to find an appropriate dosage for your particular needs.

A job situation can always be modified to improve safety, if the people involved are willing to do so. But if management refuses to protect workers, the risk of injury—not just from chemicals—is very high. When industrial workers are exposed to high levels of solvents, their functioning can be impaired, which increases the risk of accident. The number of industrial accidents and injuries caused by human error as a consequence of neurotoxic interference has not been measured, but it's an important consideration, since about 40 million industrial workers are regularly exposed to significant levels of neurotoxic chemicals.[1]

The governmental agency designed to regulate occupational safety is the Occupational Safety and Health Administration (OSHA). To contact them about safety violations, locate the OSHA office in your state. The number for the Washington, D.C. headquarters is (202) 219-8031. They can send an industrial hygienist to investigate a job site.

The National Institute of Occupational Safety and Health (NIOSH, at 800-35-NIOSH) investigates chemical injuries from unusual chemicals or chemicals that were not previously recognized as dangerous. They can perform a health hazard evaluation if they receive one request from management or a union, or three requests from individual employees. Labor unions can effectively protect employees by demanding better ventilation or reduced exposure time. Unions could also help their members by increasing education about neurotoxicity.

Sometimes people are ashamed to admit that a toxic chemical is affecting them. Certainly some symptoms are more private than others. After all, most people would not be embarrassed to report a rash, but they would be embarrassed to admit to irritability, forgetfulness, or an inability to maintain an erection.

When neurotoxic chemicals are affecting one worker, other people are probably being affected, too. The person who has the courage to come forward can initiate safety changes that protect other employees from injuries.

OFFICE WORK

On an ever-increasing basis, office workers are reporting health problems from chemical exposures in buildings. These types of injuries have been labeled sick building syndrome. Early chemical injuries from "sick buildings" were not taken seriously. Office workers, who were primarily women, were accused of "mass hysteria" or "mass psychogenic illness."[2] As this health hazard has increased, however, it's being taken more seriously. NIOSH reports that since buildings were better insulated or "tightened" in the 1970s, requests for investigations of sick building syndrome have increased from 6 percent of the agency's volume in 1970 to 75 percent in 1995.[3]

Most cases of sick building syndrome occur in buildings with windows that can't be opened. When windows are not a source of fresh air, the entire building is dependent on the ventilation system. If the system is poorly designed, if the outside vents are closed, if the vents are located near a source of contaminated air, or if toxic fumes generated inside the building are recirculated through the building, people can be seriously injured by breathing the accumulation of chemical fumes.

In one office, the fresh air intake was improperly located next to a parking lot. A parked, running vehicle next to the intake point was able to circulate diesel fumes throughout the entire building.

Sometimes the air intake vents are closed to save money on heating or cooling costs. When outside vents are closed, the air inside the building is continually recirculated. As people breathe in oxygen and exhale carbon dioxide, oxygen can be depleted. The oxygen needs to be replenished and the carbon dioxide needs to be diluted with fresh outside air. The more people there are in a building, the higher the demand for fresh air.

When reconstruction, painting, new carpeting, or other work occurs in a tight building, poor ventilation can recirculate the neurotoxic fumes. Sometimes the neurotoxic chemicals that are recirculated are regularly used at a workplace. For example, copy machines and strong cleaning chemicals are used in many offices; powerful disinfectants and anesthesia are used in many hospitals.

Effective managers will want to remedy immediately an unhealthy working environment to prevent a loss of productivity. Prudent building owners will want to keep occupants healthy to prevent loss of occupancy or future lawsuits.

What can you do to combat sick building syndrome? As a building occupant, you may want to contact maintenance and request that the fresh air intake in the building be increased. Or there may be some type of filter near where you sit that needs to be changed—a filter in a heating unit, for example. You can slightly increase the oxygen around you by bringing plants into your work space. Some plants, such as chrysanthemums, are particularly effective at detoxifying formaldehyde and other chemicals.

Another option is to buy an air filter with an activated charcoal filter (see chapter 18). If several people in the same area are being affected, they may want to purchase an air filter together. Although a good filter is not cheap, it may be less costly than missed work days, medical bills, or having to leave the job. You can also purchase an air filter for your car to reduce exposure to exhaust fumes while commuting to work.

OTHER WORK SITUATIONS

If you're able to control the materials you work with, be sure to select less toxic and nontoxic products. If you're a painter, for example, using no-VOC paints will dramatically reduce your occupational exposures (see chapter 17). People who work out of their own homes need to pay attention to possible chemical hazards in their work materials and environment.

Medical offices and hospitals can improve their indoor air quality, for example, by using hydrogen peroxide instead of alcohol to sterilize instruments. Cleaning with borax instead of a chlorine bleach and with vinegar instead of ammonia will improve the indoor air quality of any building.

IN CASE OF INJURY

It is important that you use good judgment in protecting yourself from toxic exposures at the worksite wherever possible. If you believe you are experiencing neurotoxic effects from your job, keep records of dates and types of symptoms, the people you have contacted, and the steps you've taken to remedy the situation. Don't allow continual exposure in a situation that's causing neurotoxic symptoms. Early symptoms of neurotoxicity need to be taken very seriously.

Occasionally there are situations in which the neurotoxic health risk is so great that leaving the job is the best alternative. This can be a devastating decision, but sometimes you have to choose between leaving while you're still healthy or losing the job later, after you've been seriously injured.

It's easier to find a new job if you're healthy and unemployed than if you're chemically injured and unemployed. If you sustain a serious chemical injury, you may not ever return to your current level of functioning.

People with a medical diagnosis of some type of chemical injury have legal protection from the Americans with Disabilities Act of 1992. The law requires an employer to make a reasonable accommodation for someone with a disability to allow them to work. Your employer may or may not be aware of this law. To learn about it, contact an Equal Employment Opportunities Commission office.

∾

For most people, work is an important part of life. It's a source of productivity and pride. An injury that interferes with your ability to work can be devastating. If the injury is a nonvisible chemical injury, you may be tempted to deny how serious it is. A rapid and effective response, however, may limit the injury to a short, flu-like experience rather than a severe, chronic health problem.

RECALCULATING THE RISK/BENEFIT RATIO

The innocence of the dawn of the chemical age has been shattered by a trail of cancer, birth defects, illness, and dementia. No longer are environmentalists the only ones concerned about toxic pollution. Contamination of air and water, problems of waste disposal, and the increasing impact of toxins on human health are all mainstream issues.

This book has presented a small portion of the overwhelming scientific evidence pointing to health hazards associated with neurotoxins. It's clear from the existing scientific evidence that neurotoxins are a health hazard to us all. We must not wait for the industries that brought us these perils to endlessly research problems and debate over solutions while continuing to sell us more of their neurotoxic products.

You now have knowledge about how neurotoxic chemicals actually affect your body and the warning signs of neurotoxicity. This knowledge can increase your control over your health and help you protect yourself from a chemical injury. You also have an overview of how to reduce neurotoxins in your home and in your life. We've focused on the use of chemicals in the home, because that's the environment over which you have direct control. However we need to do much more as a society. We need laws regulating industrial production and waste disposal. While these larger changes will take time, you don't have to wait to start detoxifying your home.

When industry and governmental agencies make decisions about the use of toxic chemicals, they use a risk/benefit ratio. This book was designed so that you could recalculate the risk/benefit ratio of neurotoxic chemicals for yourself. In most situations, neurotoxins can easily be replaced with less toxic or nontoxic alternatives. You can eliminate unwanted pests, clean your home, use cosmetics, and eat foods you like without exposure to neurotoxins.

In the final analysis, every time you choose to use a natural, non-polluting product in place of a neurotoxin, you are choosing a healthier life for yourself and for all of our children.

What you've read is disturbing, but it's truthful information about the pervasiveness of neurotoxic chemicals in our society and how much these poisons can affect our lives. Learning the truth about neurotoxic chemicals does not create the problem, it begins the solution. It's the truth that can set us free.

Specialty Mail-Order Products

Adzorbstar the Molecular
Adsorber
produced by: CYA Products, Inc.
211 Robbins Lane
Syosset, NY 11791
(516) 681-9394

Aireox Brand Air Filters
sold by: Aireox Research Corp.
11004 Hole Ave.
Riverside, CA 92505
(909) 689-2781

Aller-X Air Filters
(and Electo-Static Panel Filters)
sold by: Allergy-Asthma Shopper
P.O. Box 239
Fate, TX 75132
(800) 447-1100

Coast Filtration Water Filters
(Reverse Osmosis)*
142 Viking Ave.
Brea, CA 92621
(714) 990-4602

The Living Source
(Cosmetics and a wide variety of
nontoxic products and filters)
P.O. Box 20155
Waco, TX 76702
(817) 776-4878

Nigra Enterprises
(Discount air and water filters)
5699 Kanan Rd.
Agoura, CA 91301
(818) 889-6877

*For local Reverse Osmosis Water Filter producers and distributors, consult your
yellow pages.

Organic Food Cooperatives

Blooming Prairie Natural Foods	(800) 328-8241
Blooming Prairie Warehouse	(800) 323-2131
Federation of Ohio River Co-Ops	(614) 861-2667
Hudson Valley Federation of Food Co-Ops	(914) 437-5400
North East Co-Ops	(802) 257-5856
North Farm Cooperatives	(608) 241-2667
Ozark Co-Ops	(501) 521-4920
Tucson Co-Op Warehouse	(800) 350-2667

SELECT BIBLIOGRAPHY

Anderson, Alan. "Neurotoxic Follies," *Psychology Today*. July, 1982: 30-42.

Annau, Zoltan. *Neurobehavioral Toxicology*. Baltimore, Md.: The Johns Hopkins University Press, 1986.

Ashford, Nicholas and Miller, Claudia. *Chemical Exposures*. New York: Van Nostrand Reinhold, 1991.

Aspelin, Arnold, Grube, Arthur, and Torla, Robert. *Pesticides Industry Sales and Usage: 1990-1991 Market Estimates*. Environmental Protection Agency Office of Pesticides and Toxic Substances (H-7503W), Fall 1992.

Blaylock, Russell. *Excitotoxins: The Taste that Kills*. Santa Fe, N. Mex.: Health Press, 1994.

Brown, Michael. *The Toxic Cloud*. New York: Harper & Row, Publishers, 1987.

Chemicals in Progress. United States Environmental Protection Agency, Office of Pollution Prevention and Toxics, EPA-745-N-94-001, Spring 1994.

Dadd, Debra Lynn. *Nontoxic, Natural, and Earthwise*. New York: St. Martin's Press, 1990.

Doull, John, Klaassen, Curtis and Amdur, Mary. *Casarett and Doull's Toxicology: The Basic Science of Poisons*, Second Edition. New York: Macmillan, 1980.

Johnson, Barry. *Prevention of Neurotoxic Illness in Working Populations.* New York: John Wiley and Sons, 1987.

Konner, Melvin. *Medicine at the Crossroads.* New York: Pantheon Books, 1993.

Lifton, Bernice. *Bug Busters.* Garden City Park, N.Y.: Avery Publishing Group, Inc., 1991.

National Research Council. *Alternative Agriculture.* Washington, D.C.: National Academy Press, 1989.

National Research Council. *Toxicity Testing, Strategies to Determine Needs and Priorities.* Washington, D.C.: National Academy Press, 1984.

New Chemicals Program. United States Environmental Protection Agency, Office of Pollution Prevention and Toxics, EPA-734-F-95-001.

Olney, John. "Excitotoxic Food Additives—Relevance of Animal Studies to Human Safety." *Neurobehavioral Toxicology and Teratology* 6, 1984: 455-462.

Rapp, Doris. *Is This Your Child? Discovering and Treating Unrecognized Allergies.* New York: William Morrow and Company, Inc., 1991.

Roberts, H. J. *Aspartame (NutraSweet™) Is It Safe?* Philadelphia, Penn.: The Charles Press, Publishers, Inc., 1990.

Singer, Raymond. *Neurotoxicity Guidebook.* New York: Van Nostrand Reinhold, 1990.

Stone, Richard. "Zeroing in on Brain Toxins," *Science* 255, 1992: 1063.

Weiss, Bernard. "Behavioral Toxicology and Environmental Health Science," *American Psychologist*, November 1983: 1174.

Women's Health Research and the Environment: Findings of National and Regional Roundtable Meetings, Society for the Advancement of Women's Health Research. (For a copy of the report, call 202-223-8224.)

Notes

Chapter One: Is This Book for You?

1. *New Chemicals Program,* United States Environmental Protection Agency, Office of Pollution Prevention and Toxics, EPA-734-F-95-001, May 1995, p. 13.

Chapter Two: Symptoms of a Chemical Injury

1. This list is a composite based on numerous studies and reports including: Raymond Singer, *Neurotoxicity Guidebook* (New York: Van Nostrand Reinhold, 1990), pp. 3-8; W. Kent Anger and Barry Johnson, "Chemicals Affecting Behavior," *Neurotoxicity of Industrial and Commercial Chemicals,* ed. J. L. O'Donoghue (Boca Raton, Fl.: CRC Press, 1985), pp. 51-148; Barry Johnson, *Prevention of Neurotoxic Illness in Working Populations* (New York: John Wiley and Sons, 1987), and research conducted by the author and William J. Flanagan.
2. W. J. Hayes, *Pesticides Studied in Man* (Baltimore, Md.: Williams and Wilkins, 1982), p. 232.
3. Hayes, p. 357.
4. H. J. Roberts, *Aspartame (NutraSweet®), Is It Safe?* (Philadelphia, Pa.: The Charles Press, Publishers, Inc., 1990), pp. 95-99.
5. Singer, p. 6.
6. Roberts, p. 112.
7. Alan Anderson, "Neurotoxic Follies," *Psychology Today,* July 1982, pp. 30-42.
8. Singer, p. 30.
9. Hayes, pp. 393, 358.
10. Russell Blaylock, *Excitotoxins: The Taste that Kills* (Santa Fe, N. Mex.: Health Press, 1994), p. 35.

11. Roberts, pp. 128-138.
12. Megan Hicks, "NutraSweet . . . Too Good to Be True?" *General Aviation News*, July 31, 1989, pp. 6-7.
13. Singer, p. 7.
14. Anderson, p. 34.
15. Nicholas Ashford and Claudia Miller, *Chemical Exposures* (New York: Van Nostrand Reinhold, 1991), pp. 16-17.
16. *Women's Health Research and the Environment: Findings of National and Regional Roundtable Meetings*, Society for the Advancement of Women's Health Research, pp. 6-8 (for copy of the report, call 202-223-8224); and Ashford and Miller, pp. 173-175.
17. Bernard Weiss, "Behavioral Toxicology and Environmental Health Science," *American Psychologist*, November 1983, p. 1174.

Chapter Three: How Chemicals Affect Your Nervous System
1. Neil Carlson, *Physiology of Behavior*, third edition (Boston, Mass.: Allyn and Bacon, Inc., 1986), p. 69.
2. Arthur Guyton, *Textbook of Medical Physiology*, eighth edition (Philadelphia, Pa.: W. B. Sanders Company, 1991), p. 83.
3. K. Bulloch, T. Damavandy, and M. Padamchian, "Characterization of Choline O-acetyltransferase (ChAT) in the BALB/C Mouse spleen" *International Journal of Neuroscience* 76 (1994), pp. 141-149.
4. Carlson, pp. 629-635.

Chapter Four: Neurotoxins and the Disease Process
1. Raymond Singer, *Neurotoxicity Guidebook* (New York: Van Nostrand Reinhold, 1990), p. 32.
2. Neil Carlson, *Physiology of Behavior*, third edition (Boston, Mass.: Allyn and Bacon, Inc., 1986), pp. 630-631.
3. Singer, pp. 30-32.
4. Peter Spencer and Patricia Butterfield, "Environmental Agents and Parkinson's Disease," ed. Jonas Ellenberg, William Koller, and J. William Langston, *Etiology of Parkinson's Disease* (New York: Marcel Dekker Inc., 1995), pp. 319-365.
5. Geoffrey Cowley and Rebecca Crandall, "Bad Water, Faulty Genes: Closing in on the Causes of Parkinson's Disease," *Newsweek*, September 3, 1990, p. 73.
6. Spencer and Butterfield, pp. 348-349.
7. Singer, p. 8.
8. Singer, p. 6.
9. David Larson, *Mayo Clinic Family Health Book* (New York: William Morrow and Company, Inc., 1990), p. 283.
10. Barry Johnson, *Prevention of Neurotoxic Illness in Working Populations* (New York: John Wiley and Sons, 1987), p. 141.
11. Nicholas Ashford and Claudia Miller, *Chemical Exposures* (New York: Van Nostrand Reinhold, 1991), pp. 173-175; and *Women's Health Research and the Environment: Findings of National and Regional Roundtable Meetings*,

Society for the Advancement of Women's Health Research, pp. 8-10.

12. *Women's Health Research*, pp. 13-15.

13. Leszek Hahn, Reinhard Kloiber, Murray Vimy, Yoshimi Takahashi, and Fritz Lorscheider, "Dental 'Silver' Tooth Fillings: A Source of Mercury Exposure Revealed By Whole-Body Image Scan and Tissue Analysis," *The FASEB Journal*, 3 (1989), pp. 2641-2646.

14. *Women's Health Research*, pp. 6-8.

15. R. Ader, D. Felten, and N. Cohen, *Psychoneuroimmunology* (San Diego, Calif.: Academic Press, 1991).

16. D. L. Felten, K. D. Ackerman, S. J. Wiegand, and S. Y. Felten, "Noradrenergic Sympathetic Innervation of the Spleen: I. Nerve Fibers Associate with Lymphocytes and Macrophages in Specific Compartments of the Splenic White Pulp," *Journal of Neuroscience Research* 18 (1987), pp. 28-36; S. Y. Felten, D. L. Felten, D. L. Bellinger, S. L. Carlson, K. D. Ackerman, K. S. Madden, J. A. Olschowka, and S. Livnat, "Noradrenergic Sympathetic Innervation of Lymphoid Organs," *Progress in Allergy* 43 (1988), pp. 14-36; and K. D. Ackerman, S. Y. Felten, D. L. Bellinger, S. Livnat and D. L. Felten, "Noradrenergic Sympathetic Innervation of Spleen and Lymph Nodes in Relation to Specific Cellular Compartments," *Progress in Immunology* 6 (1987), pp. 588-600.

17. H. Besedovsky, E. Sorkin, D. Felix and H. Haas, "Hypothalamic Changes During the Immune Response," *European Journal of Immunology* 7 (1977), pp. 323-325.

18. R. J. Cross, W. H. Brooks, T. L. Roszman and W. R. Markesbery, "Hypothalamic-Immune Interactions: Effect of Hypophysectomy on Neuroimmunomodulation," *Journal of the Neurological Sciences* 53 (1982), pp. 557-566.

19. Ashford and Miller, p. 98; and R. Sharma, *Immunologic Considerations in Toxicology*, volumes I and II (Boca Raton, Fla.: CRC Press, 1981).

20. P. R. McConnachie and Arthur Zahalsky, "Immune Alterations in Humans Exposed to the Termiticide Technical Chlordane," *Archives of Environmental Health* 47 (1992), pp. 295-301.

21. Hahn, Kloiber, Vimy, Takahashi, and Lorscheider, pp. 2641-2646.

22. National Institute of Health, *Lupus*, National Institute of Arthritis and Musculoskeletal and Skin Diseases Information Package, BW 6/93 AR96 (Bethesda, Md.: National Institute of Health, 1995), p. 2.

23. M. Cutolo, A. Sulli, B. Seriolo, S. Accardo, and A. T. Masi, "Estrogens, the Immune Response, and Autoimmunity," *Clinical and Experimental Rheumatology* 13 (1995), pp. 217-226.; and S. A. Ahmed, N. Talal, and P. Christadoss, "Genetic Regulation of Testosterone-Induced Immune Suppression," *Cellular Immunology* 104, 1987, pp. 91-98.

24. Arthur Guyton, *Textbook of Medical Physiology*, eighth edition (Philadelphia, Pa.: W.B. Sanders Company, 1991), p. 715.

25. Ashford and Miller, pp. 173-174.

26. *Issues and Challenges in Environmental Health*, Department of Health and Human Services Public Health Service, National Institute of Health, NIH Publication No. 87-861, p. 9.

Chapter Five: How Chemicals Interact in Your Body

1. P. R. McConnachie, Arthur Zahalsky, "Immune Alterations in Humans Exposed to the Termiticide Technical Chlordane," *Archives of Environmental Health* 47 (1992), pp. 296-297.
2. Jenna Roberts and Ellen Silbergeld, "Pregnancy, Lactation, and Menopause: How Physiology and Gender Affect the Toxicity of Chemicals," *The Mount Sinai Journal of Medicine* 62 (1995), pp. 343-355.
3. W. J. Hayes, *Pesticides Studied in Man* (Baltimore, Md.: Williams and Wilkins, 1982), p. 315.

Chapter Six: The Route Chemicals Take Through Your Body

1. Arthur Guyton, *Textbook of Medical Physiology*, eighth edition (Philadelphia, Pa.: W. B. Sanders Company, 1991), p. 3.
2. John Doull, Curtis Klaassen, and Mary Amdur, *Casarett and Doull's Toxicology: The Basic Science of Poisons*, second edition (New York: Macmillan, 1980), p. 38.
3. Guyton, p. 415.
4. Doull, Klaassen, and Amdur, p. 41.
5. Doull, Klaassen, and Amdur, p. 60.
6. Joseph Rodricks, *Calculated Risks* (New York: Cambridge University Press, 1992), pp. 34-35.
7. Doull, Klaassen, and Amdur, p. 43.
8. W. J. Hayes, *Pesticides Studied in Man* (Baltimore, Md.: Williams and Wilkins, 1982), p. 227.

Chapter Seven: Neurotoxicity in Children

1. Zoltan Annau and Christine Eccles, "Prenatal Exposure," ed. Zoltan Annau, *Neurobehavioral Toxicology* (Baltimore, Md.: The Johns Hopkins University Press, 1986), pp. 154-155.
2. Annau and Eccles, p. 155.
3. H. A. Tilson, G. J. Davis, J. A. McLachlan, and G. W. Lucier, "The Effects of Polychlorinated Biphenyls Given Prenatally on the Neurobehavioral Development of Mice," *Environmental Research* 18 (1979), pp. 466-474.
4. Herbert Needleman, "Epidemiological Studies," ed. Zoltan Annau, *Neurobehavioral Toxicology* (Baltimore, Md.: The Johns Hopkins University Press, 1986), pp. 285-286.
5. Annau and Eccles, pp. 153-169.
6. J. E. Storm, J. L. Hart, and R. F. Smith, "Behavior in Mice After Pre- and Postnatal Exposure to Arochlor 1254," *Neurobehavioral Toxicology and Teratology* 3 (1981), pp. 5-9.
7. Needleman, p. 282.
8. Doris Rapp, *Is This Your Child? Discovering and Treating Unrecognized Allergies* (New York: William Morrow and Company, Inc., 1991).

Chapter Eight: Why Is Neurotoxicity Usually Undetected?

1. World Health Organization, "Principles and Methods for the Assessment of Neurotoxicity Associated with Exposure to Chemicals," *Environmental Health*

Criteria 60 (Geneva, 1986), as quoted by Raymond Singer, *Neurotoxicity Guidebook* (New York: Van Nostrand Reinhold, 1990), p. 9.

2. John Olney, "Excitotoxic Food Additives—Relevance of Animal Studies to Human Safety," *Neurobehavioral Toxicology and Teratology* 6 (1984), pp. 455-462.

3. World Health Organization, as quoted by J. E. Davies, "Neurotoxic Concerns of Human Pesticide Exposure," *American Journal of Industrial Medicine* 18 (1990), pp. 327-331.

4. Arnold Aspelin, Arthur Grube and Robert Torla, *Pesticides Industry Sales and Usage: 1990-1991 Market Estimates*, Environmental Protection Agency Office of Pesticides and Toxic Substances (H-7503W), Fall 1992, p. 1.

5. K. Mountain, B. Monninger, and M. Walker, *Pesticide Education for Health Professionals Research Project Report* (Austin, Tex.: Texas Rural Health Field Services, 1982).

6. Debra Lynn Dadd, *Nontoxic, Natural, and Earthwise* (New York: St. Martin's Press, 1990), pp. 163-165.

7. *New Chemicals Program,* United States Environmental Protection Agency, Office of Pollution Prevention and Toxics, EPA-734-F-95-001.

8. Raymond Singer, *Neurotoxicity Guidebook* (New York: Van Nostrand Reinhold, 1990), pp. 34-36.

9. Singer, p. 21.

10. *Chemicals in Progress Bulletin,* Environmental Protection Agency, Office of Pollution Prevention and Toxics, EPA-745-N-94-001 (Spring 1994), pp. 1-2, 8.

11. Nicholas Ashford and Claudia Miller, *Chemical Exposures* (New York: Van Nostrand Reinhold, 1991), p. 70.

12. *Chronology—EPA and Its Professionals' Union Involvement with Carpet,* provided by National Federation of Federal Employees, Local 2050.

13. Rosalind Anderson, personal interview, December 11, 1995, used by permission.

14. *Chronology—EPA and Its Professionals' Union Involvement with Carpet,* p. 7.

15. *Chronology—EPA and Its Professionals' Union Involvement with Carpet,* p. 7.

16. *Chronology—EPA and Its Professionals' Union Involvement with Carpet,* p. 4.

17. Richard Stone, "Zeroing in on Brain Toxins," *Science* 255 (1992), p. 1063.

18. P. R. McConnachie and Arthur Zahalsky, "Immune Alterations in Humans Exposed to the Termiticide Technical Chlordane," *Archives of Environmental Health*, 1990 47 (1992), pp. 295-301.

19. John Doull, Curtis Klaassen, and Mary Amdur, *Casarett and Doull's Toxicology: The Basic Science of Poisons*, second edition (New York: Macmillan, 1980), p. 11.

20. Doull, Klaassen, and Amdur, p. 9.

21. Doull, Klaassen, and Amdur, p. 9.

22. Bernard Weiss, "Behavioral Toxicology and Environmental Health Science," *American Psychologist*, November 1983, pp. 1174-1186.

23. Doull, Klaassen, and Amdur, p. 12.

24. Doull, Klaassen, and Amdur, p. 19.
25. Joseph Rodricks, *Calculated Risks* (New York: Cambridge University Press, 1992), pp. 63-64.
26. Bernard Weiss, "Emerging Challenges to Behavioral Toxicology," ed. Zoltan Annau, *Neurobehavioral Toxicology* (Baltimore, Md.: The Johns Hopkins University Press, 1986), p. 2.
27. Doull, Klaassen, and Amdur, p. 23.
28. Doull, Klaassen, and Amdur, p. 67.
29. W. J. Hayes, *Pesticides Studied in Man* (Baltimore, Md.: Williams and Wilkins, 1982), p. 411.
30. Russell Blaylock, *Excitotoxins: The Taste that Kills* (Santa Fe, N. Mex.: Health Press, 1994), p. 53.
31. Doull, Klaassen, and Amdur, p. 14.
32. Nicholas Ashford and Claudia Miller, *Chemical Exposures* (New York: Van Nostrand Reinhold, 1991), pp. 106-107.
33. Doull, Klaassen, and Amdur, p. 72.
34. Ashford and Miller.
35. Rodricks, pp. 213-214.
36. National Research Council, *Toxicity Testing, Strategies to Determine Needs and Priorities* (Washington, D.C.: National Academy Press, 1984), as quoted by Nicholas Ashford and Claudia Miller, *Chemical Exposures* (New York: Van Nostrand Reinhold, 1991), pp. 61-62.
37. Alan Anderson, "Neurotoxic Follies," *Psychology Today*, July 1982, p. 34.
38. *Pesticide Fact Sheet,* United States Environmental Protection Agency, Office of Pesticides and Toxic Substances, Office of Pesticide Programs (TS-766C), Fact Sheet Number 152, January 1988.
39. Doull, Klaassen, and Amdur, p. 12.
40. H. J. Roberts, *Aspartame (NutraSweet®), Is It Safe?* (Philadelphia, Pa.: The Charles Press, Publishers, Inc., 1990), p. 29.
41. Michael Brown, *The Toxic Cloud* (New York: Harper & Row, 1987), pp. 40-41.
42. Russell Blaylock, *Excitotoxins: The Taste that Kills* (Santa Fe, N. Mex.: Health Press, 1994), pp. 200-201.
43. Roberts, pp. 242-243.

Chapter Nine: Creating a Nontoxic Home
1. Lance Wallace, "VOCs and the Environment and Public Health—Exposure," ed. H. J. Bloemen and J. Burn, *Chemistry and Analysis of Volatile Organic Compounds in the Environment* (Glasgow, Scotland: Blackie Academic and Professional, 1993), pp. 1-24.
2. Rosalind Anderson, personal interview, December 11, 1995, used by permission.

Chapter Ten: Nontoxic Housecleaning
1. Raymond Singer, *Neurotoxicity Guidebook* (New York: Van Nostrand Reinhold, 1990), p. 150.
2. James Marks and Vincent DeLeo, *Contact and Occupational Dermatology*

(St. Louis, Mo.: Mosby Year Book, 1992), p. 145.
3. Debra Lynn Dadd, *Nontoxic, Natural, and Earthwise* (New York: St. Martin's Press, 1990), pp. 151-152.
4. Dadd, pp. 148-149.
5. Dadd, pp. 148-149.
6. Dadd, pp. 155-156.
7. Dadd, pp. 156-157.
8. Dadd, p. 149.
9. Rosalind Anderson, personal interview, December 11, 1995, used by permission.

Chapter Eleven: Nontoxic Pest Control
1. W. J. Hayes, *Pesticides Studied in Man* (Baltimore, Md.: Williams and Wilkins, 1982), p. 302.
2. Hayes, p. 302.
3. Raymond Singer, *Neurotoxicity Guidebook* (New York: Van Nostrand Reinhold, 1990), p. 188.
4. Singer, p. 188.
5. Singer, p. 189.
6. Hayes, pp. 284-435.
7. Hayes, pp. 436-462.
8. Hayes, pp. 172-283.
9. Hayes, pp. 333, 386.
10. Hayes, pp. 379-384.
11. Hayes, p. 399.
12. Hayes, p. 436.
13. Hayes, p. 448.
14. Singer, p. 22.
15. National Research Council, *An Assessment of the Health Risks of Seven Pesticides Used for Termite Control* (Washington, D.C.: National Academy Press, 1982), as quoted in Singer, p. 164.
16. Singer, pp. 160-166.
17. Singer, p. 21.
18. Arnold Aspelin, Arthur Grube, and Robert Torla, *Pesticides Industry Sales and Usage: 1990-1991 Market Estimates*, Environmental Protection Agency Office of Pesticides and Toxic Substances (H-7503W), Fall 1992, p. 1.
19. Jeffrey Johnson, "Roaches I Have Known," *Environmental Action*, March-April 1986, p. 16; and William Curry, personal interview, 1989, used by permission.
20. Bernice Lifton, *Bug Busters* (Garden City Park, N.Y.: Avery Publishing Group, Inc., 1991), pp. 203-208.
21. Debra Lynn Dadd, *Nontoxic, Natural, and Earthwise* (New York: St. Martin's Press, 1990), p. 171.
22. Singer, p. 191.
23. Lifton, p. 130.
24. Lifton, pp. 123-131; and Dadd, pp. 280-281.
25. National Research Council, *Alternative Agriculture* (Washington, D.C.:

National Academy Press, 1989), p. 103.
26. Dadd, pp. 170-171.
27. Dadd, p. 172.
28. Dadd, p. 169; and Lifton, pp. 101-117.
29. Lifton, pp. 85-92; and Dadd, p. 168.
30. Singer, p. 164.
31. Lifton, pp. 169-186; and Dadd, pp. 172-173.
32. Lifton, pp. 185-186.
33. Bio-Integral Resource Center (BIRC) produces quarterly publications on least toxic pest control for professionals and the general public. They can be contacted at (510)524-2567.

Chapter Twelve: Nontoxic Personal Products and Cosmetics
1. National Research Council, *Toxicity Testing, Strategies to Determine Needs and Priorities* (Washington, D.C.: National Academy Press, 1984), as quoted by Nicholas Ashford and Claudia Miller, *Chemical Exposures* (New York: Van Nostrand Reinhold, 1991) pp. 61-62.
2. *Cosmetics Handbook*, Industry Activities Staff (HFS-565), Center for Food Safety and Applied Nutrition/FDA, 1994, title page.
3. Robert Calkin and J. Stephan Jellinek, *Perfumery* (New York: John Wiley and Sons, Inc., 1994), pp. 181-186; Leslie Stewart, "Patch Testing to Cosmetics and Topical Drugs," *American Journal of Contact Dermatitis* 7 (1996), pp. 53-55; and Debra Lynn Dadd, *Nontoxic, Natural, and Earthwise* (New York: St. Martin's Press, 1990), p. 174.
4. James Marks and Vincent DeLeo, *Contact and Occupational Dermatology* (St. Louis, Mo.: Mosby Year Book, 1992), p. 145.
5. Marks and DeLeo, p. 146.
6. Stewart, p. 54.
7. Dadd, pp. 197-198.
8. Lance Wallace, "VOCs and the Environment and Public Health—Exposure," ed. H. J. Bloemen and J. Burn, *Chemistry and Analysis of Volatile Organic Compounds in the Environment* (Glasgow, Scotland: Blackie Academic and Professional, 1993), pp. 1-24.
9. Dadd, p. 251.

Chapter Thirteen: Toxin-Free Food
1. National Research Council, *Alternative Agriculture* (Washington, D.C.: National Academy Press, 1989), pp. 49-50.
2. Bernard Weiss, "Emerging Challenges to Behavioral Toxicology," ed. Zoltan Annau, *Neurobehavioral Toxicology* (Baltimore, Md.: The Johns Hopkins University Press, 1986), p. 12.
3. Arnold Aspelin, Arthur Grube, and Robert Torla, *Pesticides Industry Sales and Usage: 1990-1991 Market Estimates*, Environmental Protection Agency Office of Pesticides and Toxic Substances (H-7503W), Fall 1992, pp. 1-2.
4. National Research Council, *Toxicity Testing, Strategies to Determine Needs and Priorities* (Washington, D.C.: National Academy Press, 1984), as quoted by Nicholas Ashford and Claudia Miller, *Chemical Exposures* (New York: Van

Nostrand Reinhold, 1991), pp. 61-62.
5. *Alternative Agriculture*, p. 126.
6. *Alternative Agriculture*, p. 127.
7. Raymond Singer, *Neurotoxicity Guidebook* (New York: Van Nostrand Reinhold, 1990), pp. 19-23.
8. W. J. Hayes, *Pesticides Studied in Man* (Baltimore, Md.: Williams and Wilkins, 1982), p. 399.
9. Singer, p. 34.
10. Russell Blaylock, *Excitotoxins: The Taste that Kills* (Santa Fe, N. Mex.: Health Press, 1994), p. 226.
11. H. J. Roberts, *Aspartame (NutraSweet®), Is It Safe?* (Philadelphia, Pa.: The Charles Press, Publishers, Inc., 1990), pp. 33-35.
12. Roberts, p. 36.
13. James Freeman, "Aspartame Alert," *Flying Safety*, May 1992, pp. 20-21.
14. Roberts, pp. 136-138.
15. Blaylock, p. 211.
16. Roberts, pp. 241-242.
17. Roberts, p. 241.
18. Roberts, pp. 225-226.
19. Roberts, p. 226.
20. Blaylock, p. 213.
21. Roberts, pp. 67-139.
22. Roberts, pp. 39-40.
23. Blaylock, p. 66.
24. Roberts, pp. 176-180.
25. Blaylock, pp. 223-224.
26. Ashford and Miller, pp. 61-62.
27. Debra Lynn Dadd, *Nontoxic, Natural, and Earthwise* (New York: St. Martin's Press, 1990), p. 300.
28. Katherine Rowe and Kenneth Rowe, "Synthetic Food Coloring and Behavior: A Dose Response Effect in a Double-Blind, Placebo-Controlled, Repeated-Measures Study," *The Journal of Pediatrics* 125 (1994), pp. 691-698.
29. Dadd, p. 302.
30. Rowe and Rowe, "Synthetic Food Coloring and Behavior," pp. 691-698; Bonnie Kaplan, Jane McNicol, Richard Conte, and H. K. Moghadam, "Dietary Replacement in Preschool-Aged Hyperactive Boys," *Pediatrics* 83 (1989), pp. 7-17; and Marvin Boris and Francine Mandel, "Foods and Additives Are Common Causes of the Attention Deficit Hyperactive Disorder in Children," *Annals of Allergy* 72 (1994), pp. 462-468.
31. W. Kent Anger, "Workplace Exposures," ed. Zoltan Annau, *Neurobehavioral Toxicology* (Baltimore, Md.: The Johns Hopkins University Press, 1986), p. 332.
32. Roberts, p. 150.

Chapter Fourteen: Choices in Medicine
1. Melvin Konner, *Medicine at the Crossroads* (New York: Pantheon, 1993), pp. 62-63.
2. "History of Aspirin," Bayer Consumer Care Division, in "20th Century

Miracle Drug: From Pain Killer to Life Saver: Aspirin Reigns Supreme." (For copy, call 800-331-4536.)
3. "History of Aspirin," Bayer Consumer Care Division.
4. "Herbal Roulette," *Consumer Reports*, November 1995, pp. 698-705.
5. Bernard Weiss, "Behavioral Toxicology and Environmental Health Science," *American Psychologist*, November 1983, pp. 1175-1178.
6. Richard McNerney and John McNerney, "Mercury Contamination in the Dental Office," *New York State Dental Journal* 45 (1979), pp. 457-458.
7. J. E. Abraham, C. W. Svare, and C. W. Frank, "The Effect of Dental Amalgam Restorations on Blood Mercury Levels," *Journal of Dental Research* 63 (1984), pp. 71-73, quoted by David Eggleston and Magnus Nylander, "Correlation of Dental Amalgam with Mercury in Brain Tissue," *Journal of Prosthetic Dentistry* 58 (1987), pp. 704-707.
8. Eggleston and Nylander, pp. 704-707.
9. Leszek Hahn, Reinhard Kloiber, Murray Vimy, Yoshimi Takahashi, and Fritz Lorscheider, "Dental 'Silver' Tooth Fillings: A Source of Mercury Exposure Revealed by Whole-Body Image Scan and Tissue Analysis," *The FASEB Journal* 3 (1989), pp. 2641-2646.
10. Bill Wolfe, "Mercury-Silver Fillings: An Historical Perspective and Update," *Health Consciousness* 13 (1992), pp. 84-85.

Chapter Sixteen: Nontoxic Lawns and Gardens
1. National Research Council, *Alternative Agriculture* (Washington, D.C.: National Academy Press, 1989), p. 44.
2. John Doull, Curtis Klaassen, and Mary Amdur, *Casarett and Doull's Toxicology: The Basic Science of Poisons*, second edition (New York: Macmillan, 1980), p. 389.
3. Raymond Singer, *Neurotoxicity Guidebook* (New York: Van Nostrand Reinhold, 1990), p. 23.
4. National Research Council, pp. 104-105.
5. National Research Council, pp. 122-123.
6. National Research Council, pp. 162-164.
7. National Research Council, pp. 122-123.
8. Kenneth Geluso, J. Scott Altenbach and Ronald Kerbo, *Bats of Carlsbad Caverns National Park* (Carlsbad Caverns Natural History Association, 1987), pp. 1-29.
9. National Research Council, pp. 123-124.
10. National Research Council, pp. 123-124.
11. Barbara Ellis and Fern Bradley, *The Organic Gardener's Handbook of Natural Insect and Disease Control* (Emmaus, Pa.: Rodale Press, 1992), pp. 132-133; and Stuart Franklin, *Building a Healthy Lawn* (Pownal, Vt.: Garden Way, 1988), pp. 11-154.
12. Franklin, p. 128.
13. Personal interview with Troy Myers at Lambert's Landscapes in Dallas, Texas, on 5/20/96, used by permission.
14. *Organic Gardening*, April 1995, p. 84.
15. Jeff Cox and the Editors of Rodale's Organic Gardening Magazine, *How to*

Grow Vegetables Organically (Emmaus, Pa.: Rodale Press, 1988), p. 69.
16. Ellis and Bradley, p. 10.
17. National Research Council, pp. 108, 145.
18. National Research Council, pp. 126-127.
19. Personal interview with Troy Myers at Lambert's Landscapes in Dallas, Texas, on 5/20/96, used by permission.

Chapter Seventeen: Low-Toxicity Home Improvement and Construction
 1. Nicholas Ashford and Claudia Miller, *Chemical Exposures* (New York: Van Nostrand Reinhold, 1991), p. 65.
 2. Raymond Singer, *Neurotoxicity Guidebook* (New York: Van Nostrand Reinhold, 1990), p. 147-148, 166-176.
 3. Debra Lynn Dadd, *Nontoxic, Natural, and Earthwise* (New York: St. Martin's Press, 1990), p. 277.
 4. J. William Hirzy and Rufus Morison, "Carpet/4-Phenylcyclohexene Toxicity: The EPA Headquarters Case," ed. B. J. Garrick and W. C. Gekler, *The Analysis, Communication, and Perception of Risk* (New York: Plenum Press, 1991), p. 53.
 5. Dadd, p. 274.
 6. Dadd, pp. 274-275.

Chapter Eighteen: Air and Water Filters
 1. *Chemicals in Progress Bulletin*, Environmental Protection Agency, Office of Pollution Prevention and Toxics, EPA-745-N-94-001 (Spring 1994), p. 2.
 2. Michael Brown, *The Toxic Cloud* (New York: Harper & Row, 1987).
 3. *Chemicals in Progress Bulletin*, pp. 1-2, 8.
 4. National Research Council, *Alternative Agriculture* (Washington, D.C.: National Academy Press, 1989), pp. 104-105.
 5. Kenneth Cantor, "Water Chlorination, Mutagenicity, and Cancer Epidemiology," *American Journal of Public Health* 84 (1994), pp. 1211-1213.
 6. Bette Hileman, "Fluoridation of Water," *Chemical and Engineering News*, August 1, 1988, pp. 34-36.
 7. C. H. Turner, M. P. Akhter, and R. P. Heaney, "The Effects of Fluoridated Water on Bone Strength," *Journal of Orthopaedic Research* 10 (1992), pp. 581-587.
 8. Hileman, p. 41.
 9. Hileman, pp. 29-32.
10. Hileman, pp. 26-42.

Chapter Nineteen: Managing Toxins at Work
 1. Raymond Singer, *Neurotoxicity Guidebook* (New York: Van Nostrand Reinhold, 1990), p. 15.
 2. Nicholas Ashford and Claudia Miller, *Chemical Exposures* (New York: Van Nostrand Reinhold, 1991), p. 113.
 3. According to the NIOSH recorded message on indoor air quality, fall 1995— (800)35-NIOSH.

INDEX

AUTHOR

CYNTHIA FINCHER received her PhD and MS in health psychology and behavioral medicine from the University of North Texas. She attended the University of California at Santa Barbara where she received her BA and multiple academic honors, including the psychology department award for academic excellence.

She has published original research focused on the effects of neurotoxic exposures on brain functioning. In 1993 she developed a seminar, which was the basis of *Healthy Living in a Toxic World*. Her goal is to make information about healthy lifestyle changes accessible and achievable for everyone.

Dr. Fincher is currently in clinical practice, and she is pursuing future research and writing projects.

What do I believe about money

What my attitude

Did I feel Tony should take care
of my wants

if I spend more than I make

lack of confidence

Lord show me how to overcome